WESTSIDE BARBELL
BOOK OF SQUAT AND DEADLIFT

by Louie Simmons

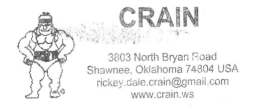

CRAIN

3803 North Bryan Road
Shawnee, Oklahoma 74804 USA
rickey.dale.crain@gmail.com
www.crain.ws

Westside Barbell Book of Squat and Deadlift
by Louie Simmons

Writer: Louie Simmons
Editor: Sakari Selkäinaho
Photographs: Doris Simmons
Covers and layout: Lasse Arkela, 4Life.fi
Printer: Action Printing, WI
Copyright © Westside Barbell, Louie Simmons 2011

Disclaimer
The author and publisher of this material are not responsible in any
manner whatsoever for any injury that may occur through following
the instructions contained in this material. The activities may be too
strenuous or dangerous for some people. The readers should always
consult a physican before engaging in them.

TABLE OF CONTENTS

DEDICATION

I would first like to thank the Culver City California Westside Barbell Club for their innovative training methods even in the 1960s. It was the powerlifting articles written by Bill "Peanuts" West and George Frenn in the old Muscle Power Builder that sold me on box squatting. Those articles helped me, first, reach the top ten in the squat and total and kept me in the top ten throughout my 30-year career.

Many others have inspired or helped me out along the way. I was amazed by Paul Anderson and his colossal strength. Unfortunately, I never saw Paul in person, but when I saw him on tape for the first time, the hair stood up on my neck. It was like seeing an alien or Bigfoot. I just can't explain it.

George Crawford was the first to give me advice on squatting. He was light years ahead of his time. Jack Barnes from Arizona was unreal in all the lifts, but his squat was out of this world. In 1973, I made 630 lbs at a body weight of 181 lbs, but Jack was the king at 710 lbs at a body weight of 181 lbs without any gear.

John Kanter, Jon Cole, Don Reinhoudt, and Larry Pacifico all inspired me in the early years. Dr. Fred Hatfield was next to come. Fred thought out of the box with compensatory acceleration training (CAT) and plyometrics.

I will never forget Mike Bridges back in 1977. This kid came up to me and said, "I'm Mike, and I'm going to break a world record." I wished him luck, and he did just what he said he would do. In my opinion, he is the greatest powerlifter of all time. Mike had it all—strength, technique, and a limitless mind.

Many helped the Westside plan, but Matt Dimel put it into full use, setting the world record in the super heavyweight division with a 1010-lb squat. Chuck Vogelpohl is a Westsider who personifies squatting, setting world records at body weights of 220, 242, and 275 with 1150 lbs. That exceeded the 308-lb body weight record at the time.

Now the deadlifters. Vince Anello from Cleveland, Ohio, could defy gravity. My old buddy, Danny Wohleber, pulled the first 900-lb deadlift at a body weight of 275 lbs in 1982.

Lamar Gant was a phenomenon at a body weight of 123 and 132 lbs. At the world championships in Dayton, Ohio, Precious McKenzie pulled 556 lbs to tie the world record at a body weight of 123 lbs, and though everyone thought it iced the championship, Lamar called 622 lbs. That's 66 lbs over the existing world record. He just came out and pulled it. That was the first and only standing ovation I've ever seen at a power meet. Lamar was a true gentleman as well.

Bob Peoples of Tennessee was a real inspiration to my training. He was using advanced systems in the 1940s that are complicated for many of today's lifters to comprehend.

Ed Coan pulled 901 lbs at a body weight of 220 lbs. I can't even comprehend the feat. Ed is the strongest man I've ever seen. His ability to handle heavy weights was off the charts in both squatting and deadlifting.

When I saw Alexander Kuscher pull 793 at a body weight of 165 lbs at the WPO meet in Columbus, Ohio, I nearly passed out. In the words of my dear friend Eskil Thomasson, some say the weights weren't real, but they were!

When I saw Garry Franks and Andy Bolton pull back to back 900-lb deadlifts, it was truly an honor to be there. And speaking of Andy Bolton, I never thought I would witness a 1000-lb deadlift after Danny pulled that first 900 in 1982. But in upper state New York, Andy was the first to pull over 1000 lbs—1003 lbs to be exact. I saw it. I bit my lip to see if I was still alive, and I was.

I have a tattoo on my arm that says, "Born 1947–died never." Now, I'm going to have to keep that promise because I know there are more great things to see.

Now the scientists. Yes, I must thank the scientists like Mel Siff, who was very instrumental in helping me apply science to sports. Others include (in no particular order)

Ben Tabachnik, PhD; Vladimir Zatsiorsky, PhD, for his tireless work; Michael Yessis, PhD, for his contribution to advancing strength sports; Thomas Kurz; Tudor O. Bompa and A.N.Mededev for work on periodization; P. Komi for his numerous writings; R. Berger, Andrzej Lasocki, Tadcsz Starzynski, and Henryk Sozansko, PhD, for their work on power development; and Y.V. Verkhosansky, the father of shock training, whose work has pushed us to constantly think. A virtual problem is one that is there but not recognized.

I would like to thank Bud Charniga, Jr., for first giving me access to "The Soviet Systems for Training" and the many college and professional coaches who have come to visit Westside, including Buddy Morris, Dave Williams, Tommy Myslinski, Johnny Parker, Joey Batson, and Bill Gillespie, who said I was his secret weapon.

I know I can't thank everyone. There are just too many.

Last but not least, it would not be possible for me to write this book and other books without the tireless help from Sakari Selkäinaho, the only man I trust with bringing forth my material to the readers. I will always be indebted. Thank you, Sakari. I'd like to thank

Diane Black for making me sound much smarter than I am by editing my articles. Thank you, Diane.

And finally, I need to thank my wife, Doris, for letting me put my ambition for strength ahead of everything else.

- Louie

From the editor

This manual is the third publication from Louie Simmons. Westside Barbell Bench Press Manual, which came out in 2009 after the long-awaited The Westside Barbell Book of Methods, was an eye-opener for many, giving hands on guidance and instructions on how bench pressing is done at Westside.

The Westside Barbell Book of Squat and Deadlift will do exactly the same. It covers the dynamic training cycles done at Westside along with everyone´s favorite maximum effort exercises.

A personal best is always an achievement and in fact the only proof for correct training. You can see what kind of training has resulted in which results. You will also notice that to achieve the same goal there are many ways. To make constant progress, training must be individually planned. The higher you go, the more individual differences there will be. Every lifter must find their own way to the top. For that purpose, this book gives a lot of useful tools.

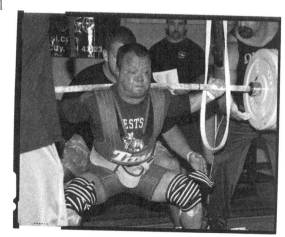

Load the bar, make your goals a reality!

- Sakari
  Selkäinaho

INTRODUCTION

Westside divides the training for the squat and deadlift into two days. Fridays are reserved for squatting and are referred to as speed days. Speed days are a cycle of a three-week wave using weights that are roughly 75–85 percent of a one rep max on a box squat. A wave of strength-speed is where weights range from 90 to slightly over 100 percent. This is also done for a three-week wave. The final phase before a meet, the circa-max phase, consists of weights ranging from 90–97 percent. This phase lasts for two weeks and ends with a new personal record on the box squat. It leads to a delayed transformation phase of one week of downloading. These waves will be thoroughly explained later.

W e do very little work under 70 percent. When barbells move at high velocities, they yield low force.

The maximal effort method is used for the second training day for the squat and deadlift (Monday). In the words of Vladamir Zatsiorsky, "Lifting maximal weights will cause the fastest muscle units to be recruited, and the maximum number of muscle units is activated. The discharge frequency of motor units is at its highest, and the activity of the muscle is synchronous."

All exercises contribute to the squat and the deadlift. A good morning will build both the squat and deadlift. A squat, especially a front squat, will raise the deadlift. A max rack deadlift will build the ability to lift a heavy squat or deadlift. How? Time under tension. However, you have to produce the maximal muscle tension it takes to perform a squat or deadlift. This system is the conjugate system, which uses exercises similar to the classical lifts to perfect form by identifying weaknesses. Our entire training system is based on the conjugate system. We aren't built the same, so a squat or deadlift will affect a particular muscle group at a lesser or greater extent depending on the individual. This can lead to either injuries or lack of progress.

After each of the two days, the repetition method is employed. The course of special exercises is constantly changed. Lifters must select five or more exercises for each major muscle group. The exercises and waves are linked, and the amount of general physical preparedness (GPP) and restoration are constantly raised and lowered.

This has been a brief overview of the Westside system. Let's go to a more precise explanation.

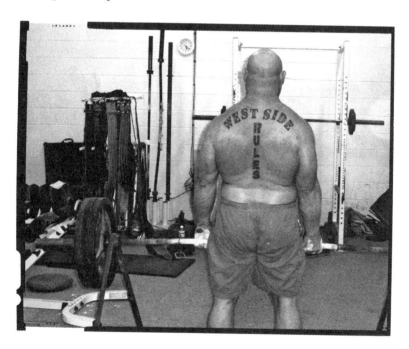

WESTSIDE STRENGTH METHODS

Westside uses the three proven methods of strength training—the dynamic method, the maximal effort method, and the repetition method.

The Dynamic Method

The dynamic method is used to increase a fast rate of force development and explosive strength. It was first used to replace a max effort workout when needed. Because it is impossible to display maximal force in fast movements against small and intermediate loads, this method won't build or increase maximal strength. Refer to the Hill equation of muscle contraction for more information and to learn the physics behind this.

The dynamic method is followed by 2–4 special exercises.

Maximal Effort Method

This method is superior for both intramuscular and intermuscular coordination. Vladamir Zatsiorsky said that the muscles and central nervous system only adapt to the load placed on them, meaning if you want to lift heavy weights, you must train with heavy weights. The maximal effort method will bring about the largest strength gains.

At Westside, our maximal effort day is based on the Bulgarian system. We max out each week. It may not be an all-time max, but it's an all-out max on that particular day. We know that training with weights at 90 percent and above for three weeks will cause our training to regress due to muscular and central nervous system breakdown. So to avoid this, we switch the major bar exercise each week. This is known as the conjugate system.

The max effort workout should occur 72 hours after speed day. At Westside, our speed day is Sunday so our max effort day is Wednesday. This gives us ten days to rest from heavy bench pressing for a contest. Speed day is seven days from a contest. The weights are light, and we reduce the sets to six. The special exercises are reduced as well. This works perfectly for the delayed transformation of the training load.

The weights lifted on max effort day should be done with little emotion to avoid stress. If you reach a high level of emotion too often, you'll max out. If this happens when you're training, it will interfere with competition.

The Repetition Method

Repetitions are how we control intensity and volume. Westside never performs high reps in the squat, bench, or deadlift in training. We only perform two reps (squat), three reps (bench), and one rep (deadlift) for those lifts. The high reps are reserved for lats, triceps, delts, and upper back.

When the work is performed after benching or on max effort day, this is considered hypertrophy. The number of exercises or sets and reps is dependent upon your level of preparedness, but you should perform 2–4 exercises. Switch exercises when you need to based on your mental or physical state. Introverts can get by with fewer exercises than extraverts can.

At Westside, we believe it is our duty to teach you to train yourself. After ten months, you should have a firm grasp on the system as it pertains to your training.

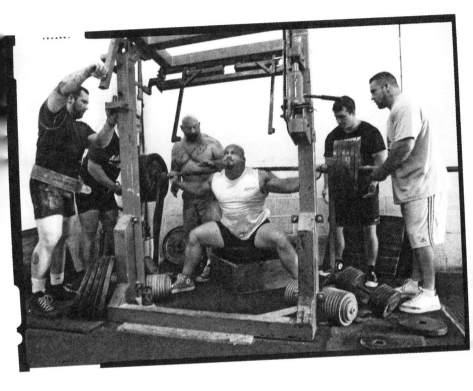

Chapter 2

THE CONJUGATE SYSTEM

The conjugate system was first scientifically introduced in 1972 in the former Soviet Union. The famed Dynamo Club with 72 highly qualified Olympic weightlifters was used as the prototype. They were given 20–45 special exercises to choose from. After the first monthly cycle, the coaches asked the lifters for their conclusions on the training program. One lifter was satisfied and the rest wanted more exercises to choose from.

T he Westside system is the conjugate system in its entirety. We use a mix of Russian and Bulgarian combined with my own experiences, and we've developed over 90 elite lifters.

The max effort exercises are changed each week, and the reactive methods are changed as often as we see fit. The small, special exercises are changed often so that we never adapt to training. We use different gear—some strong and some not so strong. We also adjust box and pin heights each week to bring positive results.

The conjugate system uses a weekly plan, which is based on a larger plan encompassing the month and year. Max effort day is and must be connected to dynamic day. Special strength training must use exercises similar to the classical lifts, whether they are Olympic lifts or power lifts. With high level lifters, a special training system must be imposed to produce a more powerful training effect. When a lifter has already been accommodated to high results in the classical lifts, special barbell exercises must be introduced into the program. Other special strengths can be raised by using individual means and specific motor skills such as speed-strength and endurance.

I was using the conjugate method in 1970 and didn't know it. I was training by myself, and to escape boredom, I deadlifted and benched off of a wide variety of power rack pin heights. I also used five different box heights for squatting and many different bench grips. I'm sure I wasn't the first one to do this. In fact, bodybuilders use the conjugate system with or without knowing it when they train at different gyms with different equipment. For example, bodybuilders visit different gyms and do leg presses on many slightly different machines that work at different angles. I see all sports as using the conjugate method with one play leading to a different play in order to win the game or be successful. Boxers throw a punch to set up a combination or fake their opponents into a position to get hit. Everything in sports is connected in some way to the next move.

At Westside, we seldom do regular squats. Instead, we box squat 99 percent of the time. One lifter, Eskil Thomasson, squatted 804 lbs and then injured his knees. He didn't do a regular squat for five years. On his return to the platform, he made 810 lbs. In his second meet back after three more months of training, Eskil made an official 840-lb squat. Again, he didn't perform regular squats, only box squats. Another lifter, John Stafford, only deadlifted once a month yet was an 832-lb deadlifter at a body weight of 275 lbs. John did low box squats on different boxes and a wide variety of good mornings. He did some rack pulls or stood on a two- to four-inch box, but he never did any regular deadlifting until meet day.

Our top benchers only perform shirt maxes maybe once every four weeks. Instead, they max out on floor presses with bands and chains, board presses, or incline and decline bench presses, or they use cambered bars and other specialty bars. Once you can spell your name correctly, you can't spell it any better. The same goes for bar exercises. Your form will deteriorate if you don't do more difficult exercises. A box squat done correctly makes a regular squat much easier to perform. It also gives the lifter a chance to max out all year long, which is accomplished by switching a major core exercise each week on max effort day.

The Westside conjugate system almost completely eliminates the biological law of accommodation. Zatsiorsky states, "Accommodation is a decrease in the response of a biological object to a continued stimulus." Here the exercises are the stimulus. This is precisely why the Westside conjugate system is superior to all others. Many of the special workouts are for the legs, back, and abs. They are designed to improve the classical lifts using a concept known as delayed transformation.

The conjugate system has two major factors—adaptation and de-adaptation. Ben Tabachin, who invented the parachute, said, "To adapt to training is to never adapt to training." That's the Westside conjugate system at its best. The system isn't any one system, yet it is all systems combined. The work should be divided into 85 percent concentric and 15 percent eccentric.

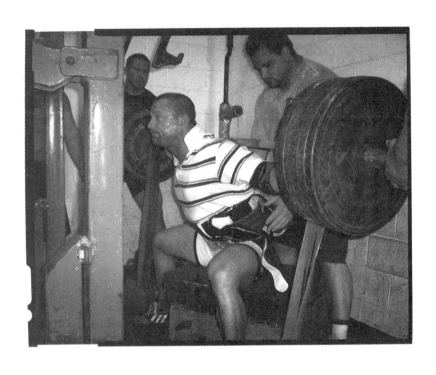

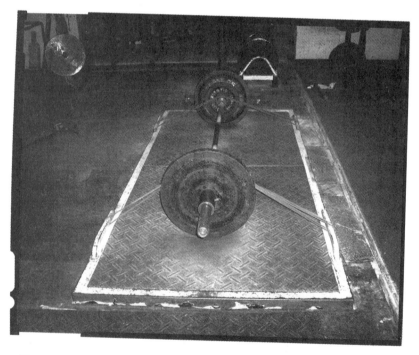

Chapter 3

ACCOMMODATING RESISTANCE

There are three primary methods to maximize weight training: accentuation (work is done at the exact angles at which maximal force is produced), peak contraction (maximal strength is developed at the weakest body position such as in the start of a pec deck), and accommodating resistance (near maximal force is developed throughout the entire range of motion (Vladamir Zatsiorsky).

Westside uses many forms of the latter—accommodating resistance—including bands, chains, and weight releasers.

The future method is used to reduce bar deceleration and produce an overspeed eccentric, which then produces a virtual force effect. This is known as the contrast method. Here the weight is constantly different at the top of the lift than it is at the bottom. Although sometimes as much as 40 percent over a lifter's best squat was lowered, there wasn't any evidence that showed overloaded eccentrics worked in many experiments.

Chains

Chains are as old as time. By attaching them to the barbell in a correct manner, the chains will unload as the lifter lowers into the bottom of a squat. As the lifter rises concentrically, the chains reload to accommodate resistance. There has to be a perfect weight in the bottom of the lift as well as at the top. The reloading and unloading of the chains provides this. Use a three-week wave with weights ranging from 405–480 lbs for ten sets of two reps. In a meet, this setup yields an 805-lb squat for three of our lifters by adding 120 lbs of chains to the barbell. Our 1000-lb and higher squatters use as much as 300–360 lbs of chains. This method has worked since the 1990s and it still does today.

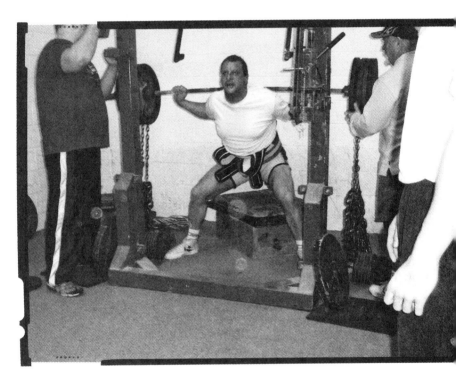

Weight Releasers

At Westside, we also use weight releasers to accommodate resistance. The Soviets used to overload a bar and have the athletes lower themselves to the bottom of the squat. At that point, spotters stripped off a predetermined amount of weight, and the athlete performed the concentric phase unassisted.

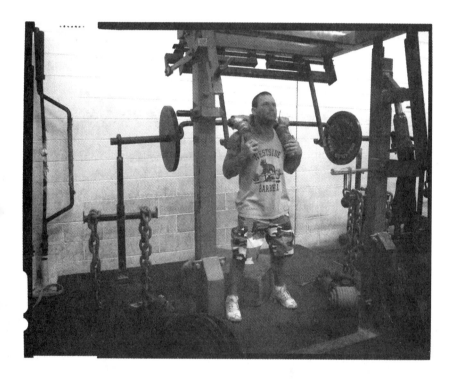

Bands

We started using bands in the mid-1990s. Bands have given us the most success to date. Many lifters think that bands only help accommodate resistance on the concentric phase, but the eccentric phase is greatly enhanced because the bands provide added speed, which causes a greater stretch reflex and Golgi tendon reflex. The bands help build great muscle size. Through many experiments, we found to within one tenth of a meter per second that the faster you go down, the faster you get up. To develop different strengths, you must adhere to a certain combination of band ratio to barbell weight. This will build tremendous jumping ability as well. This is truly accommodating resistance.

Remember, force equals mass times acceleration. It is as important on the eccentric phase as it is on the concentric phase. Newton's second law must be looked at constantly to reach a high level. His first law states that an object at rest tends to stay at rest and an object in motion tends to stay in motion in a straight line at a constant speed. To overcome a large mass at rest, a large amount of stretch reflex must be exerted. The bands work a lot like connective tissue because they stretch and contract. Westside uses many combinations of bands, chains, and weight releasers in two- or three-week waves, and then we switch to another accommodating resistance method.

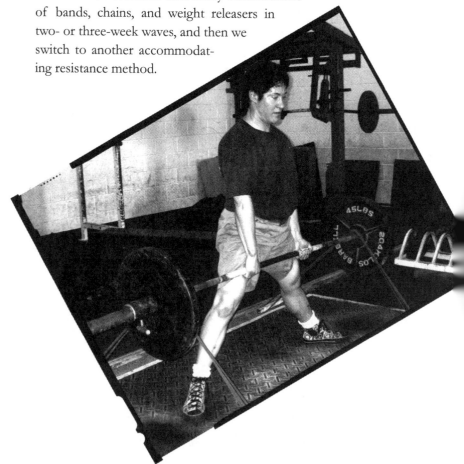

Future Method

The Soviets used the future method for many of their junior lifters. It is often used in gymnastics for tumbling. Bands are fixed at the top of the rack, and the barbell is suspended by the bands, reducing the load in the bottom of a lift. For example, a barbell held inside a set of strong bands will reduce the load from 135 lbs at lockout to zero lbs at the bottom. As the lifter lowers the bar to the bottom of the squat, the load is reduced to the amount mentioned—zero lbs. As the lifter presses the bar to lockout, the bar weight is unloaded from the bands and reloaded to the original 135 lbs.

The future method teaches optimal eccentrics by assisting the lifter in lowering the barbell. It also teaches lifters to accelerate concentrically by squatting onto foam blocks. This works much like the future method with bands. The lifter sits on the foam or lowers the barbell plates onto the foam. Once again, the lifter is learning both optimal eccentrics and acceleration. At Westside, the foam training has produced a sizable increase in muscle mass in both the upper and lower body.

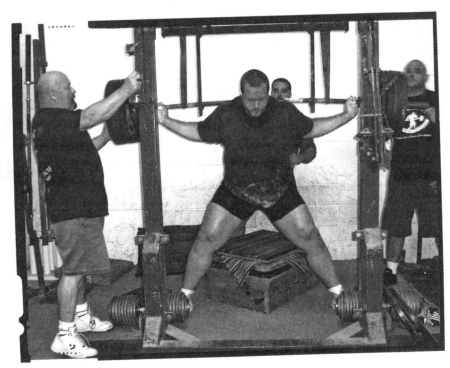

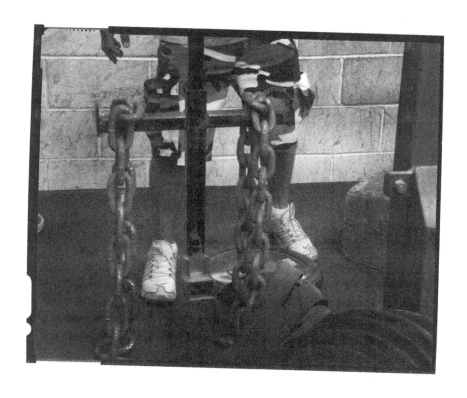

Chapter 4

MAXIMAL EFFORT METHOD

The most superior training method for improving both intra-muscular and intermuscular coordination as well as top absolute strength is the maximal effort method. The maximal effort method uses aspects of the Bulgarian system and the Soviet system. The Bulgarian system has lifters maxing out on each workout for that day, although they may not necessarily get an all-time max for a lift. The Soviet system only counts all-time maxes. Both systems use Olympic-based lifting.

At Westside, we max out every Monday and Wednesday. We squat and deadlift on Mondays, and we bench on Wednesdays. Like the Bulgarians, we max out regardless of our training ability. We might not achieve an all-time record, but it's all we were capable of on that day. This means lifters who aren't close to a meet won't get PRs while lifters who are approaching a meet should make PRs.

Although the Bulgarians primarily used six main exercises, we use countless special exercises designed to build the weakness of each lifter in all three lifts. Like the Soviets, the system we find most effective is the conjugate system. A wide variety of special exercises such as good mornings, box squats, rack pulls, and many forms of squatting are constantly rotated to make training more effective and fun, which allows for a longer lifting career. If you have a longer career in any sport, you will benefit from new technology such as tracks, balls, ball fields, and in our case, supportive gear. Unlike either the Bulgarian or Soviet systems, we seldom use the competition lifts.

Our system is limited to total max singles regardless of what our level of preparedness is during the training year. The process is much like preparing for a contest in that we work up in as large of a jump as possible. The first lift is at around 90 percent and gives the lifter an estimate of how strong he is on that training day. The second lift should be at or near 100 percent (or slightly above). The third lift is for a new personal best and should be as much as the lifter can possibly get on that given day. That's a total of three lifts with the possibility of one or two new gym records or personal bests.

We do this type of training for all types of deadlifts and squats. We also do this concentrically with good mornings for no less than triples. Because all three lifts build the large muscle groups used in both the squat and deadlift, we use them to promote the competition squat or the competition deadlift. Absolute strength is measured in the time it takes to complete the task. This means a special squat will help build the deadlift and vice versa. Furthermore, good mornings will build both the squat and deadlift, depending on how they are executed.

It is commonly known that the central nervous system and the muscles adapt only to the load placed on them. Because the body's muscular system and the central nervous system adapt quickly, we do a new exercise each week to avoid accommodation. The volume is constantly being raised through special exercises for the legs, back, and abs. To lift new maxes, we must constantly raise our general physical preparedness (GPP) and use all available restoration methods. When using the maximal effort method in training, avoid high emotional stress. Save the high emotions for a contest max.

The core exercises must be close to the biomechanical parameters of the classical lifts—power or Olympic. Doctor Squat said it best—"If light weights make you strong, why not lift just light weights?" Of course we know he was right, and that's why the max effort method works best. As of January 1, 2010, we have developed 88 elite lifters. I believe our success comes from maxing out on maximum effort day even if we don't have a meet scheduled. We do this all year long.

Hill determined that the speed of movement is dependent on maximum muscular strength. Did you hear that football strength coaches? Physics states that maximum force is attained when velocity is small. Consequently, maximum velocity is attained when external resistance is near zero *(Theory and Practice of Physical Culture)*. Why do I bring this up? Do you want to be faster and stronger?

A study in *Strength and Power in Sport* by Paavo Komi showed that the greatest weightlifters in the world lifted the heaviest weights at the slowest speeds. This simply shows that it is better to have a high level of strength over a high rate of speed. I have been using this system at Westside since 1983 when Bud Charniga translated many books for me from the former Soviet Union. I started learning and talking about the books. Many have read some of the same books but haven't considered the number of lifts or the percentages that are determined with the Olympic lifts. This won't work with the power lifts.

Olympic lifts have a bar speed of 1.2 meters per second (mps) to 1.4 mps in the first pull. A second pull of 2.2 mps can be attained. Top power lifts of 0.5–0.7 mps have been achieved. Olympic lifting is primarily a speed-strength sport, and the time under tension is brief. The power lifts are quite a different story. They are mainly a strength-speed or slow strength sport. This means the training percentages are somewhat higher. However, even Olympic lifts are seldom below 70 percent.

The table below shows the breakdown of Olympic lifts by percentages of a one rep max as well as the distribution of loads. Forty-nine and a half percent of the lifts are at 75–85 percent, and 27.1 percent of the lifts are above 85 percent.

Distribution of Loads Relative to Maximum Snatch and Clean and Jerk of Qualified Lifter											
Loads (%)											
Exercise	Up to 55	55	60	65	70	75	80	85	90	95	100
Snatch	0.83	0.0	4.08	6.19	11.7	11.7	14.5	22.9	16.7	8.9	2.5
Clean & jerk	1.36	1.86	4.82	7.88	8.18	16.6	14.9	18.4	12.7	11.0	2.3
Mean data	1.09	0.96	4.45	6.99	9.91	14.1	14.7	20.7	14.7	10.0	2.4

Remember, this is based on Olympic lifts, which are much faster than power lifts. While max force production occurs at 0.4 seconds, you must maintain that until the lift is complete. As you can see in the graph, weights are used mostly at 85 percent, so we try to wave from 75 to 85 percent in three-week waves. Only 23.4 percent of the lifts are performed at 70 percent or below. This table was based on 780 highly qualified weightlifters (A. D. Ermakov and N. S. Atanasov, 1975).

As stated, the Westside maximal effort method is a combination of the Bulgarian system, the former Soviet Union system, and my 43 years of powerlifting with over 88 elite powerlifters. The Soviet Union was very vast geographically, which led to many different body types and ethnic groups. Because of this, they used many different exercises to develop the shortcomings of their lifters. Sounds just like Westside.

In Pavvo Komi's book, *Strength and Power in Sport*, Arkady Vorobyev states that the Soviet team did 20,000 lifts—both classical and special—per year. Of those, 600 were maximal lifts (new records). The lifters were chosen for the team after they completed a three-year preparatory phase of base work, which was performed to ensure that they were suited to handle the work loads, both physically and psychologically. This is known as the "Rule of Three." The Soviet weightlifters were much more diversified than their Bulgarian counterparts.

The Soviet team did two workouts a day, which was composed of pulls, good mornings, and squats. Westside also trains two times a day. The difference is the second workout is directed toward a specific body part(s). For example, the second workout might be directed toward the low back, lats, and abs or triceps, traps, and biceps.

While the Soviet team was tremendous, the Bulgarian team was amazing. They only chose model weightlifters who fit within a specific height and weight index. Bulgaria is around the size of Ohio. Both the junior and senior national teams trained together under a few coaches led tightly by Coach Ivan Abadjiev. It was his way or the highway. If a lifter couldn't handle the stress of constantly using max or near max lifts, he was replaced. Coach Abadjiev chose to limit the training to six lifts—the power snatch, snatch, power clean, clean and jerk, front squat, and back squat. After warming up, the Bulgarian team did six max effort singles in the power snatch or snatch within 45 minutes to keep testosterone levels as high as possible. They took a 30-minute rest and then did the power clean and jerk or clean and jerk and front or back squats. This amounted to 18 near max lifts performed daily—one in the morning session, one in the afternoon, and the one in the evening. The pulls and squats were trained this way all the time. Remember, the coaches were very fastidious in who they picked for the team. They only selected lifters who could handle the stress of training like this six days a week in addition to formally structured training on good mornings and back squats. I based Westside's max effort days on this system.

Let's compare the Soviet and Bulgarian systems. The majority of the Soviets' training is centered on about 50 percent of their lifts at 75–85 percent and 20 percent of their lifts at 90–100 percent. On the other hand, the Bulgarians train mostly at 90–100 percent for their max effort lifts and 90–97 percent for their circa-max lifts. The Bulgarian system has produced the highest results in weightlifting. Why? They handle the highest average weights most often. It's that simple. Yes, they use a very select group of lifters, but their system is the best.

I had the pleasure of spending a day at Westside with a former doctor for the Bulgarian weightlifting team. He said many lifters couldn't perform the tasks asked of them. More times than not, it was the psychological stress, not the physical demands that halted their progress. I have seen the same thing at Westside. Handling weights above 90 percent for three weeks in the classical lifts can cause a lack of progress due to accommodation. At Westside, we change a max effort lift each week. We avoid staleness by doing exercises that are similar to but aren't actually the regular squat, bench press, and deadlift.

Westside has developed a system of maxing out on non-classical lifts. This allows us to eliminate the negative responses of training close to maximum competition weights. If we repeated the same lift each week, the same negative response would occur with the special lifts. However, we switch lifts every week to avoid this. Remember, the muscles and central nervous system adapt only to the load placed on them. Vladimir Zatsiorsky states that the maximal effort method brings forth the greatest strength increments plus central nervous system inhibition if it exists.

Now we know the max effort method is superior to all others. You must train at the highest average of a one rep max as often as possible. I realize this is impossible for most lifters in every workout, which is why we use the dynamic effort method. We use submaximal weights with maximal speed. Our squat training is mostly around 75–85 percent for multiple sets with briefs and a belt. Remember what Doctor Squat said? "If light weights work, why not use light weights?" But light weights don't work.

When Chuck Vogelpohl trained at Westside, he handled the heaviest average weights when he squatted and deadlifted. He was our best squatter and set world records in the 220- and 275-lb weight classes. He's now at a different gym, and at 242 lbs. Greg Panora handles the heaviest weights now at Westside. If you average the squat, bench press, and deadlift, he has dominated the 242-lb world record total. Look at

Big Iron, and I'm sure you will see the same.

Vladimir Zatsiorsky states, "It's impossible to exert a large amount of force against a small mass." Dr. Hatfield was right. The men and women who can recruit the most muscle units are the strongest. The maximal effort method does just that—allows lifters to recruit more muscle units. The next best method is the circa-max method, which uses 90–97.5 percent of weights. The circa-max method differs in that it can include multiple sets of one or two reps per set up to ten total lifts per workout (Siff). Note: The Bulgarians had great restoration methods including Jacuzzis, saunas, massages, and others at their disposal.

Weights are seldom calculated at less than 70 percent. The Soviets' and Westside's training are very similar in that the squats and pulls are mostly in the 75–85 percent range on dynamic effort day, and we're always working up to a current max on max effort day. Remember, some supportive gear is almost always worn. On dynamic bench day, the percent is very low at 40–50 percent, but there isn't any gear worn, and there are always bands or chains on the bar. When the dynamic method is used, the muscles are contracted very quickly and forcefully. I personally experience more soreness on speed day.

The dynamic method was developed to replace a max effort day for those who couldn't handle two max effort workouts per week. This helped me recover from a bad back injury in the early years. I couldn't handle two max effort lower and upper body workouts per week, which is why we changed over to the dynamic method. We made one day a quick day, not a light day, and kept the heavy day, or max effort day, because we knew the heaviest weight lifted in the gym would materialize in meet records if done correctly.

There are many methods of training that are used on both max effort and speed day. It is very important to change the core and special exercises frequently. In addition, it is vital that you change the bar speed by using bands, chains, weight releasers, heavy weight, and light weight. Monitor your intensity zones properly. For example, a 400-lb squatter should be doing the same amount of work proportionally as a 900-lb squatter. Just when your body has all the answers, you have to change the questions.

Chapter 5

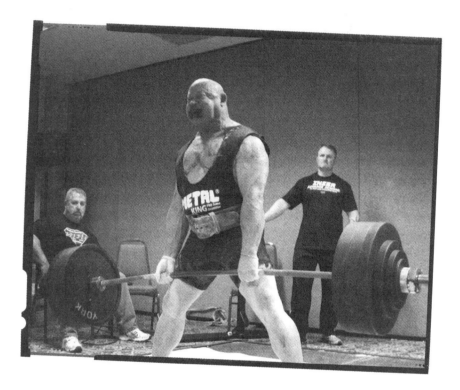

TWENTY MAXIMAL EFFORT WORKOUTS

Workout #1

- Max out with Buffalo bar on 10-inch box

- Glute ham raises with weight, 5 sets

- Reverse hypers, 3 sets with a strap, 3 sets on the ultra reverse hyper with the roller

- Stretch

Workout #2

- Concentric good morning with safety squat bar, work up to max single

- Belt squats, 6 sets of 6 reps with moderate weight

- Lat pull downs, 8 sets of 8–12 reps

- Reverse hypers, 3 sets on a strap, 3 sets with heavy

- Hanging leg raises, 5 sets

- Stretch

Workout #3

- Low pin deadlift, work up to max single

- One leg squats, 5 sets of 10 reps while holding dumbbells

- Dumbbell rows, 4 sets of 8 reps each side

- Sled pulls, 6 trips of 200 feet with moderate weight walking forward

- Reverse hypers, 2 sets with a strap, 2 sets with the roller

- Stand up abs, 5 sets

- Stretch

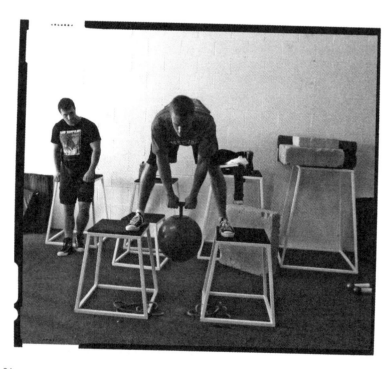

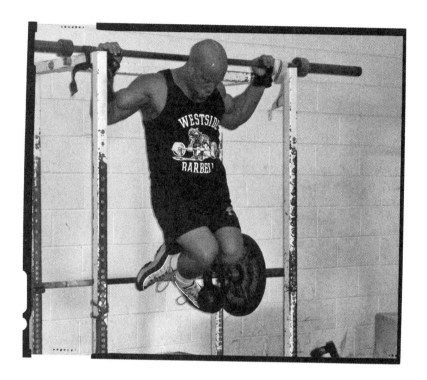

Workout #4

- Deadlift standing on 2-inch box for max single

- Kettlebell deadlifts standing on bench, 3 sets of 20 reps with weight range from 88–195 lbs

- Reverse hypers, 2 sets with straps, 3 sets with the roller

- Barbell rows with curl grip, 6 sets

- Bent leg sit-ups with weight, 5 sets

- Stretch

Workout #5

- Ultra-wide sumo deadlift for max single

- Belt squats sitting into the foam box, 6 sets of 5 reps

- Chin-ups with weight, 5 sets of 6 reps

- Reverse hypers with a strap, 6 sets

- Leg raises with weight, 5 sets of 10 reps

- Stretch

Workout #6

- Very heavy sled pulls, 6 pulls of 200 feet walking forward, 6 pulls walking backward

- 45-Degree back raises, 6 sets of 6 reps with heavy weight

- Barbell rows, 5 sets of 8 reps

- Walk 0.5 miles with 20-lb ankle weights, lifting legs high for abdominal and hip development

- Stretch

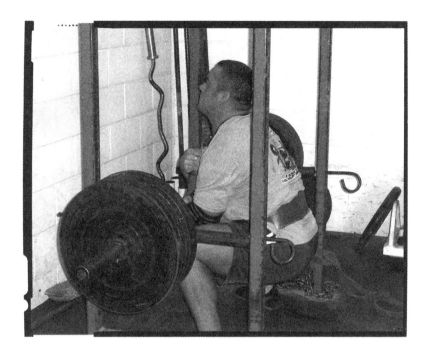

Workout #7

- Safety squat bar squat on 10-inch box for a 5RM

- Walking good mornings with Safety squat bar for 250 feet

- Back raises, 6 sets of 15 reps with moderate to light weight

- Reverse hypers with a strap, 3 sets

- Stand up abs, 6 sets of 10–12 reps

- Stretch

Workout #8

- Zercher lifts on floor, work up to a 3RM; reduce weight and do 2 sets of 5 reps

- Belt squats with light weight, 5 sets of 10 reps

- Chest supported rows, 4 sets of 8 reps

- Reverse hypers, 3 sets of 8 reps with a strap, 3 sets of 8 reps with the roller

- Straight leg sit–ups, 6 sets 8 reps

- Stretch

Workout #9

- Power clean for max single; then power snatch for max single

- Heavy sled pulls, 8 trips of 200 feet backward; close grip pull downs

- Heavy dumbbell rows, 8 sets of 6 reps

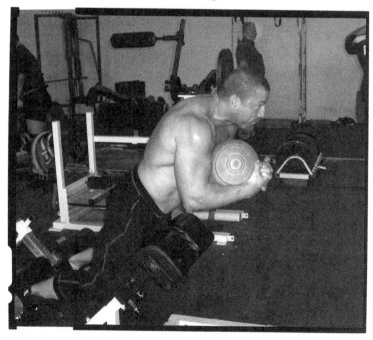

- Hanging leg raises, 5 sets of 6 reps with weight

- Stretch

Workout #10

- Rack pulls with 350 lbs band tension plus weight, 3 reps per set when possible and then go for max single

- Chin-ups with weight, 6 sets of 5 reps

- Reverse hypers, 3 sets with a strap, 3 sets with the roller

- Straight leg sit-ups, 5–6 sets with weight

- Stretch

Workout #11

- Belt squat without box, work up to 5RM

- Good mornings with approximately 70%, 4 sets of 6 reps

- Dumbbell rows, 6 sets of 6 reps on each side

- Glute ham raises, 5 sets of 6 reps per set with resistance

- Reverse hypers, 2 sets with a strap, 2 sets with the roller

- Crunches, high reps

- Stretch

Workout #12

- Fourteen-inch cambered bar Good mornings, lower weight onto foam blocks for 3RM

- Glute ham raises, 6 sets of 6 reps with weight

- Back raises with heavy weight

- Reverse hypers with a strap, 5 sets

- Straight leg sit-ups, 6 sets of 10 reps with weight

- Stretch

Workout #13

- Front squat, work up to 5RM and then work back down in sets of 8 reps

- Back raises with bar held in hands, 6 sets

- Chest-supported rows, 6 sets of 6 reps as heavy as possible

- Reverse hypers, 2 sets with straps, 2 with the roller

- Stand up abs

- Stretch

Workout #14

- Zercher squats off of 10-inch box after warm up, sets of 3 reps

- Light sled pulls, 10 trips of 200 feet forward

- Chin-ups with weight

- Reverse hypers, 2 sets with straps, 2 sets with the roller

- Hanging leg raises, 5 sets of 10 reps with light weight

- Stretch

Workout #15

- Band deadlifts, work up to max single with approximately 350 lbs of bands plus weight

- Belt squats, 5 sets of 8 reps

- Barbell rows, 4 sets of 8 reps with wide grip

- Reverse hypers with a strap, 4 sets

- Straight leg sit-ups with weight

- Stretch

Workout #16

- Safety squat bar with large amount of chains, work up to max single

- Chest-supported rows, 6 sets of 8 reps

- Kettlebell deadlifts, 3 sets of 20 reps with 88–154 lbs

- Reverse hypers, 2 sets with straps, 2 sets with the roller

- Stand up abs

- Stretch

Workout #17

- Sumo rack pulls, use low pins 2–6 inches off floor with plates

- Front squats, 6 sets of 6 reps off high box 2 inches above parallel

- Dumbbell rows, 5 sets of 8 reps each sideReverse hypers, 2 sets with straps, 2 sets with the roller

- Stand up abs

- Stretch

Workout #18

- Heavy sled pulls with weight vest, max weight for 6 trips of 100 feet

- Walk 0.5 miles with 20-lb ankle weights

- Crunches with no weight

- Reverse hypers, 3 sets with the roller

- Stretch

Workout #19

- Sumo box deadlift standing on 2-inch box, work up to max single

- Light sled pulls, 6 trips of 200 feet

- Chest-supported rows

- Stand up abs with light weight, sets of at least 1 minute

- Reverse hypers, 3 sets with straps, 3 sets with the roller

- Straight leg sit-ups, 4 sets

- Stretch

Workout #20

- Concentric squat with a safety squat bar off pins (sit on box under bar, sit up straight clearing pin, relax for 2 seconds and then stand up)

- Lat pull down with wide grip, 8 sets of 10 reps

- Kettlebells deadlifts, 3 sets of 20 reps with 88–154 lbs

- Reverse hypers, 3 sets with straps, 3 sets with the roller

- Weighted leg raises, 5 sets of 6–8 reps

- Stretch

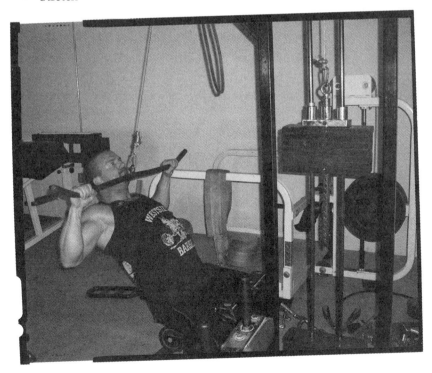

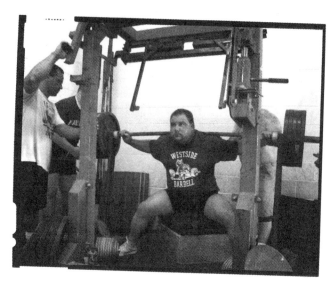

These twenty workouts can be done in any order and mixed up to your liking. Do what works for you, not what you like to do. When performing the major exercises, think about why you're performing the lift and whether it will help your squat or deadlift.

Do what works best before the contest. Some lifters need more leg work while others may need more back work. When you're worn down, do general exercises and stay away from barbell exercises. You can do small workouts 6–24 hours after restoration. Beginners should perform two extra workouts per week while advanced lifters should perform up to eight extra workouts per week.

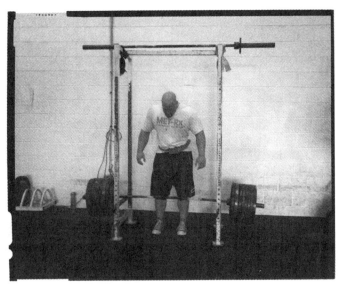

WESTSIDE MAX EFFORT FAVORITES

Matt Smith, 1160-lb squat, 850-lb deadlift

1. Suspended good mornings with the bar three feet off the floor with only the bar weight or an extra 300 lbs of chain weight

2. Lightened deadlift (Matt does singles, and his best is 820 lbs with blue bands.)

3. Safety squat bar on a low box, bar weight only or with chains or bands

Vlad Alhazov, 1250-lb squat, 925-lb deadlift

1. Regular bend over good mornings, bar weight only for a 3RM and 5RM

2. Rack pulls with the bar 2, 4, and 6 inches off the floor using bar weight or 250–350 lbs of band tension at the top

3. Low box squats using a 14-inch cambered bar or front squat harness

4. Zercher squats off of the floor or in a power rack

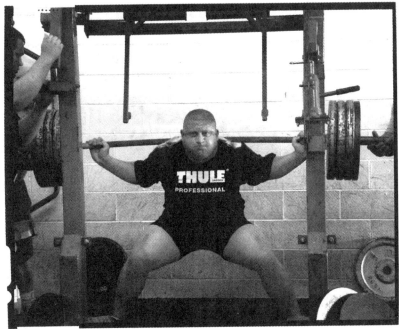

Vlad Alhazov

Tim Harold, 1010-lb squat, 855-lb deadlift

1. Safety squat bar on a low box

2. Rack pulls 2, 4, and 6 inches off the floor

3. Ultra-wide deadlifts using an Okie deadlift bar with collars on the bar before adding plates (This is the meaning of ultra-wide deadlifts; Tim is 6 feet, 7 inches.)

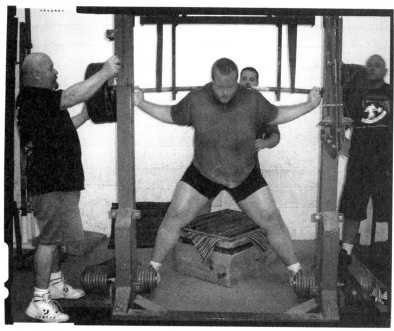

Tim Harold

Chuck Vogelpohl, 1150-lb squat, 835-lb deadlift

1. Rack pulls of all kinds with bar weight only or bar weight plus bands

2. Box deadlifts off a 2- or 4-inch box

3. Low box squats with a Safety squat bar or front squat harness

4. Zercher squats off of a low box or rack

5. Band over bar deadlifts

Mike Brown, 1074-lb squat, 804-lb deadlift

1. Foam box squats with a variety of bars using parallel and low boxes and a close and wide stance

2. Rack pulls with weights 2, 4, and 6 inches off of the floor

3. Zercher squats lifted off the floor and in the power rack

Greg Panora, 1060-lb squat, 815-lb deadlift

1. Rack pulls using bar weight only or with bands

2. Safety squat bar squats on a low box using a close and wide stance

3. Front squats and Zercher squats on a low foam box

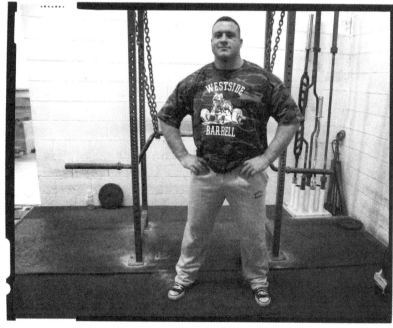

Greg Panora

Tony Bolognone, 1100-lb squat, 765-lb deadlift

1. Safety squat bar squats on a low, hard box or with foam using only bar weight or with bands

2. Rack pulls with bar weight only or with bands

3. Ultra-wide sumo deadlifts

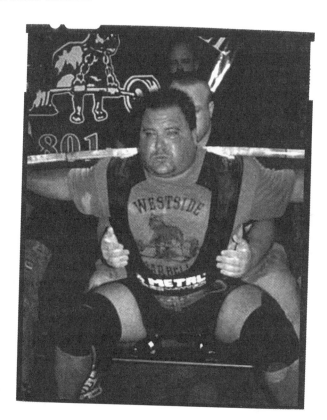

Tony Bolognone

Mike Ruggiera, 1050-lb squat, 821-lb deadlift

1. Band deadlifts off of the floor

2. Rack pulls with or without bands

3. Front squats on a low box or low box squats on foam with chains or bands added in sometimes

4. Overspeed eccentric box squats using bands and weight releasers to increase the speed on the eccentric phase

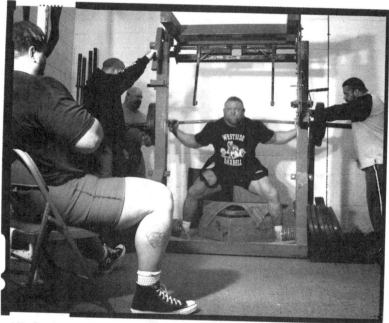

Mike Ruggiera

Matt Dimel, 1010-lb squat, 821-lb deadlift

1. Low box squats using a close and wide stance

2. Rack deadlifts with the weights 2, 4, and 6 inches off of the floor

3. Bent over good mornings

Dave Hoff, 1015-lb squat, 800-lb deadlift

1. Foam box squats at parallel and below parallel

2. Rack pulls with or without bands

3. Band pulls off of the floor with a variety of band tensions

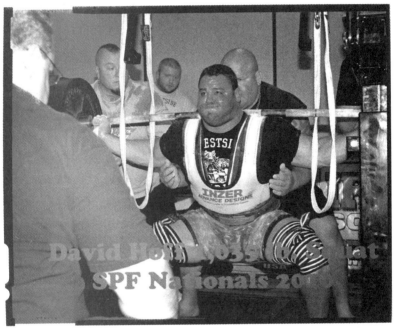

David Hoff

Luke Edwards, 1015-lb squat, 815-lb deadlift

1. Rack pulls with the weights 2, 4, and 6 inches off of the floor with or without bands

2. Zercher squats off of the floor or in a power rack with or without bands

3. Front squats on a low box with heeled shoes

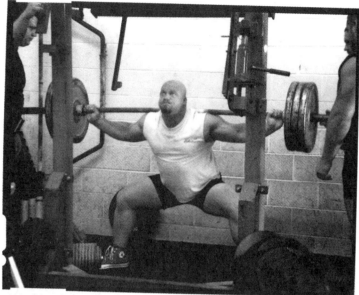

Luke Edwards

John Stafford, 947-lb squat, 832-lb deadlift

1. Rack pulls with or without bands

2. Band pull deadlifts off of the floor

3. Box deadlifts off 2- and 4-inch boxes

4. Front squats and Safety squat bar squats on a low box with or without bands.

A.J. Roberts, 1008-lb squat, 760-lb deadlift

1. Wide low box using 14-inch cambered bar, sometimes with bands

2. Rack pulls with and without bands

3. Good mornings with 2-inch and 14-inch cambered bars with chains and bands

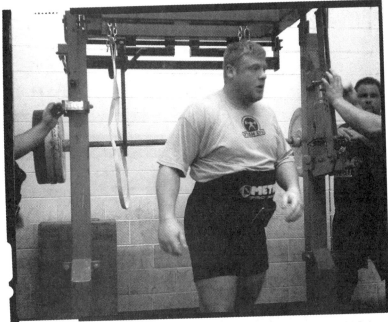

A.J. Roberts

Amy Weisberger, 590-lb squat, 500-lb deadlift

1. Front squats on a hard box with low foam

2. Good mornings of all kinds, bent over or arched back, straight or bent legs

3. Bow bar squats on a low box using a wide or close stance wearing either flat Chuck Taylors or high-heeled boots

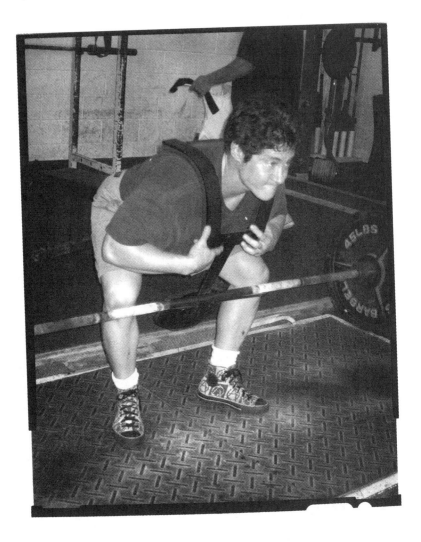

Laura Phelps, 770-lb squat, 560-lb deadlift

1. Future method with monster mini- or light bands

2. Straight or bent leg wide sumo deadlifts with or without bands

3. Close stance low box squats or front squats on foam, bar weight only or with chains or bands.

These workouts are rotated weekly to prevent accommodation. Of course, this is the conjugated system. After the max effort core lift, the lifters perform 2–4 special exercises for the low back, abdominals, and lats. These are constantly rotated whenever it's necessary.

Remember, do a workout that works for you, not what you like to do. Whatever you like the best is almost always not what works the best.

Perform lots of reverse hypers, special leg curls with ankle weights, and all types of sled pulling.

It will take about ten months for you to find what works for you individually. Once progress starts, it won't stop until you reach your full potential—if it exists.

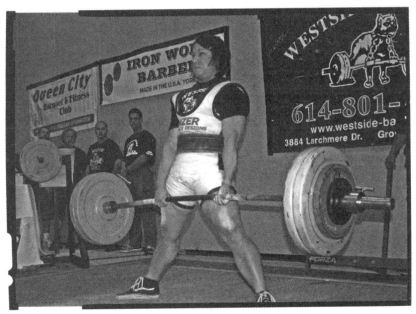

Laura Phelps

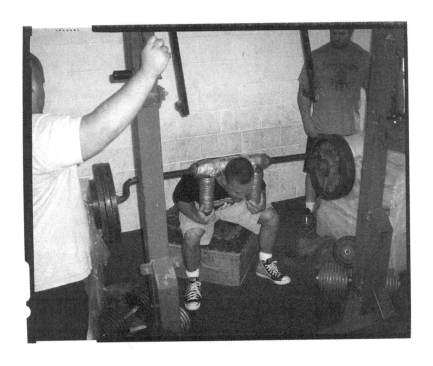

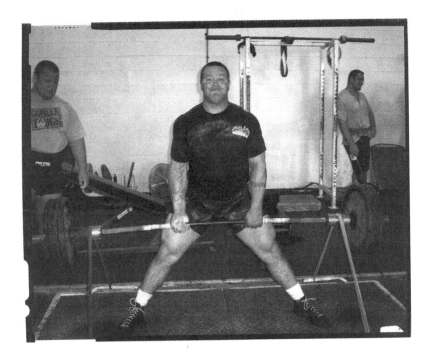

MAX EFFORT EXERCISES FOR THE SQUAT AND DEADLIFT

Max Effort Good Mornings

1. Good mornings with arched back and bent legs

2. Good mornings with rounded back and bent legs

3. Good mornings with arched back and straight legs

4. Wide stance good mornings

5. Close stance good mornings

6. Heels raised good mornings

7. Toes raised good mornings

8. Concentric good mornings

9. Good mornings with a power bar

10. Good mornings with a safety squat bar

11. Good mornings with a cambered bar

12. Good mornings with a Back Attack machine

13. Walking good mornings

14. Band good mornings

15. Seated on bench good mornings

16. Seated on floor good mornings

17. Split leg good mornings

Good mornings can be done with chains, bands, or weight releasers or any combination of the above.

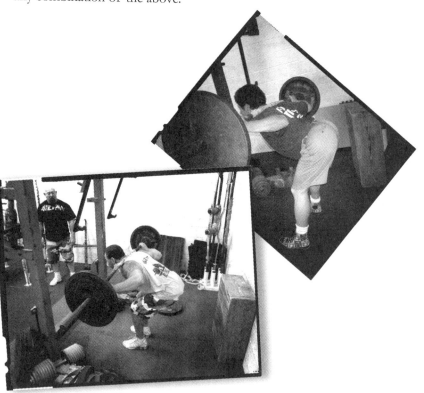

Max Effort Squats

1. Belt squats

2. Front squats

3. Zercher squats

4. Squats with a safety squat bar

5. Squats with a cambered bar

6. Squats with a Manta Ray

7. Squats with a buffalo bar

8. Incline squats

9. Decline squats

10. Weight vest squats

11. Overhead squats

12. One-leg squat sprinters or Anderson style

13. Concentric squats

14. Squats with bands, chains, or weight releasers

15. Squats on boxes or without boxes

16. Squats on boxes below parallel, at parallel, and above parallel

17. Squats with a wide to a very wide stance or a close to a very close stance

18. Leg presses

19. Lunges

20. Jumping

21. Depth jumps

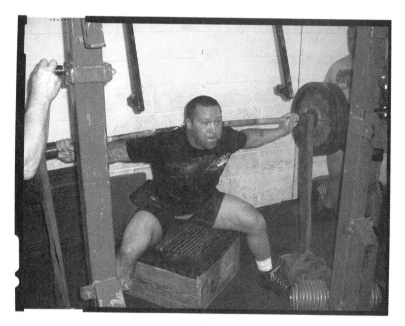

Max Effort Deadlifts

1. Straight leg deadlifts

2. Rack pin deadlifts

3. Box deadlifts

4. Sumo deadlifts

5. Conventional deadlifts

6. Band deadlifts

7. Chain deadlifts

8. Eccentric deadlifts

9. Wide grip deadlifts

10. Regular grip deadlifts

11. Reverse grip deadlifts

12. Hook grip deadlifts

13. Zercher lift deadlifts

14. Power cleans from 4 positions

15. Power snatches from 4 positions

16. Isometric deadlifts

17. Dumbbell deadlifts

18. Jefferson deadlifts

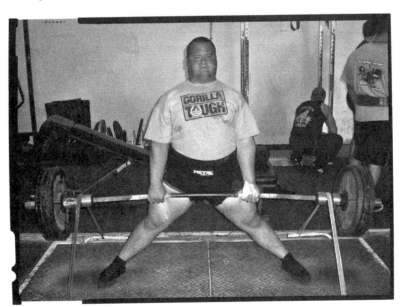

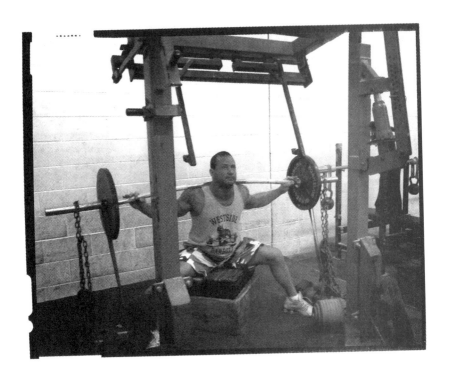

THE DYNAMIC METHOD

The dynamic method was introduced for two reasons—to improve the rate of force development and explosive strength and to replace the maximal effort workout. Many lifters can't handle max effort workouts on a constant basis. So instead they use a lower intensity workout at 75–85 percent. With the dynamic system, it is impossible to attain full maximal isometric tension of the muscles used, which is why the dynamic method isn't used for increasing maximal strength.

The dynamic method is good for extremely slow lifters. When using this method, you must use the highest attainable speed due to the relationship between force and velocity. If the velocity is high, the force production will be low. Use weights at 70–85 percent accompanied by accommodating resistance to eliminate bar deceleration. I used the dynamic method after breaking the L5 disc in my back for the second time. Because of my injuries, I had become slow. However, I was determined to push to my fullest potential. With submaximal weights of 75–85 percent for multiple sets, I became explosive again. Think about this—if you squat 1000 lbs, you must train with at least 700 lbs to produce significant force. Cut the math in half for a 500-lb max.

The dynamic method alone won't build maximal strength, which can be explained by Hill's equation for muscle contraction and supertraining.

When all three strength methods are combined—dynamic, maximal, and repetition efforts—you can increase your maximum strength.

We perform the dynamic effort method on Fridays using submaximal weights with maximal speed for up to 24 lifts. With light weight, it's impossible to obtain maximum force because of the explosive strength deficit. So with light weight, the rate of force development and explosive strength should increase when weights up to 40–70 percent are used. This day is also for the submaximal effort method, or lifting with submaximal weight, where we move loads ranging from 75 to 85 percent with maximal speed for up to 20 lifts.

Our squat day is for the circa-maximal method as well as the maximal effort method. The weights range from 90 to 97 percent of a one rep max. These loads permit a lifter to do several sets of mostly two reps (sometimes one rep per set) for a total of 4–10 lifts per workout. We duplicate a contest with one weight at close to 90 percent and one weight close to or slightly under an all-time personal record. The squat cycles are done in three-week waves, and we add weight or more band tension each week. The circa-max wave is only two weeks due to its severity. An additional week is used as a down week for delayed transformation.

The strength-speed phase lasts two weeks, and then we shift into a light dynamic wave. This is because the bar has a deceleration phase. Bands or chains must be added to the bar for accommodating resistance because the bands provide overspeed eccentrics. Don't be fooled by the total load on the bar. Whether the box is soft or hard, force equals mass times acceleration when you come into contact with it. Chains will provide accommodating resistance, while bands will provide accommodating resistance plus an overspeed eccentric, causing a virtual force effect.

Chapter 9

THE REPETITION METHOD

The repetition method is also called the repeated effort method. It is a large part of the Westside system. The repeated effort method differs only in the amount of lifts per set. Submaximal efforts are normally 2–6 reps, while the repeated method uses much higher lifts per set, sometimes as high as 30 reps per set. Choose weights that cause great fatigue. If the muscles aren't greatly fatigued, they won't be trained sufficiently. The squat and deadlift are never used for repeated efforts because this can create muscle imbalances, which can cause injuries. Instead use back raises, glute ham raises, reverse hypers, and lat and abdominal exercises with the repetition method.

We use the repeated method to not only build larger muscles but also to bring up the lagging muscle groups to eliminate muscle imbalances that cause injuries. Many times, high repetitions will teach proper muscle coordination patterns and raise muscular endurance. The repetition method is used after maximal effort and/or dynamic method day, or it can take the place of a maximal effort workout. On squat and deadlift maximal effort day, sled pulling, belt squatting, and kettlebell shrugs for high reps can be substituted. These movements are of somewhat low intensity and high volume and are directed to a precise muscle group. Be careful not to overwork any of the muscle groups.

When your body and emotions are worn out, you should have special workouts to use for recovery and to build up any lacking muscle groups.

For the advanced lifters, these workouts can be done 12–24 hours after a major workout. Remember, these workouts can be either high or low in volume. They must be planned by the lifter or coach, and they must fulfill the special needs for the lifter to succeed. Barbell curls won't help your squat, and calf raises will do little for your bench. So without a plan, you plan to fail.

Here are some examples of some small or extra repetition methods.

Workout #1

- Glute ham raises, 5 sets

- Reverse hypers, 5 sets

- Hanging leg raises, 5 sets

- Barbell rows, 5 sets

- Walk one mile with 10-lb ankle weights

Workout #2

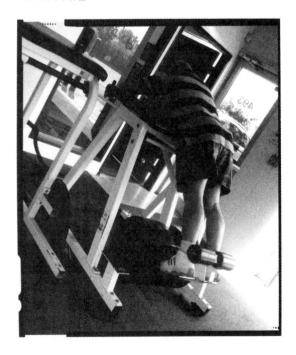

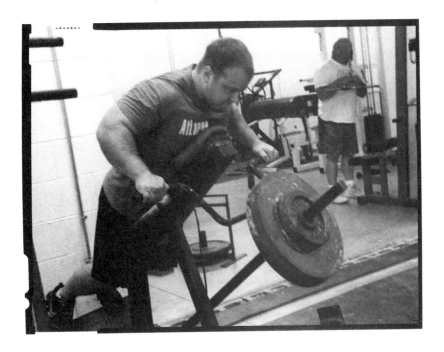

- Belt squats with a flat surface, 5 sets

- Belt squats inclined 15 degrees, 5 sets

- Belt squats declined 15 degrees, 5 sets

- Straight leg sit-ups, 5 sets

- Chest-supported rows, 5 sets

Workout #3

- Walking good mornings, 2 sets of 200 feet

- Straight leg power cleans, 5 sets

- 45-degree back raises, 5 sets

- Hanging leg raises, 5 sets

- Barbell shrugs, 5 sets

- Moderate box jumps, 5 sets

Workout #4

- Sled pulls with varying weight, 10 sets of 200 feet

- Walk 0.5 miles with 50-lb weight vest

- Dumbbell power cleans, 5 sets

- Reverse hypers, 5 sets

- Lying leg raises, 5 sets

Workout #5

- Light stiff leg deadlifts, 5 sets

- Box jumps with dumbbells, 5 sets

- Power cleans off knees, 5 sets

- Power snatches off knees, 5 sets

- Weighted sit-ups, 5 sets

Workout #6

- Front squats, 5 sets

- Lat pull downs, 5 sets

- Dumbbell shrugs, 5 sets

- Glute ham raises, 5 sets

- Reverse hypers, 5 sets

- Hanging leg raises, 5 sets

Workout #7

- Zercher squats, 5 sets

- Stiff leg deadlifts, 5 sets

- Reverse hypers, 5 sets

- Glute ham raises, 5 sets

- Box jumps with weighted vest, 5 sets

- Hanging leg raises, 5 sets

Workout #8

- Belt squats, 5 sets

- 45-degree back raises, 5 sets

- Barbell shrugs, 5 sets

- Reverse hypers, 5 sets

- Walk 1 mile with 50-lb weight vest plus 10-lb ankle weights

Workout #9

- Stiff leg power cleans, 5 sets

- Walking good mornings, 2 sets of 200 feet

- Zercher squats, 5 sets

- Chest-supported rows, 5 sets

- Reverse hypers, 5 sets

- Hanging leg raises, 5 sets

Workout #10

- Low box Manta Ray squats, 5 sets

- Stiff leg deadlifts on 4-inch box, 5 sets

- Heavy sled pulls, 6 trips for 200 feet

- Dumbbell shrugs, 5 sets

- Glute ham raises, 5 sets

In the sample workouts above, mix and match the exercises to make different combinations. The workouts should vary from very light for restoration and general physical preparedness (GPP) to very specific for a particular body part. For example, you could work the traps, hamstrings, and abdominals or lats. It is up to you to know your weaknesses and work on them to prevent injury and perfect form. These workouts can replace a max effort day workout and should occasionally lessen the mental fatigue of constantly maxing out.

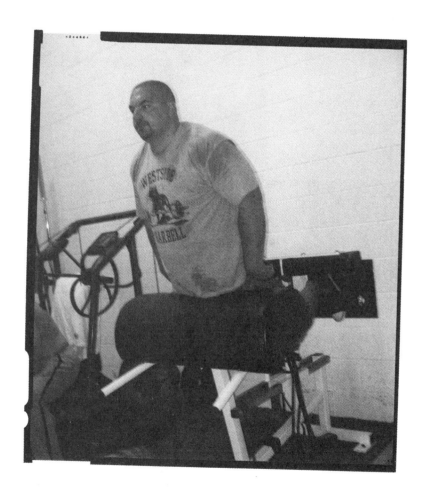

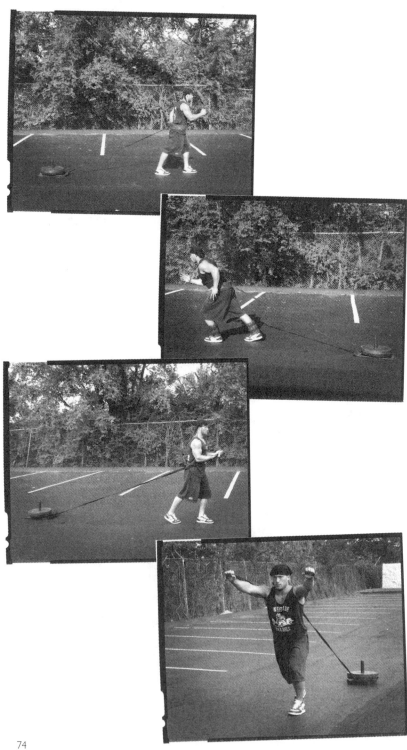

Chapter 10

HYPERTROPHY TRAINING

At Westside, we try to increase muscle mass on all training days. After the classical lifts, we work on one or more muscle groups. This is because we know that strength increases when the central nervous system is stimulated and improved. Coordination and muscular development are improved as well, providing the exercises are correct for the chosen sport.

After the barbell is retired for the day, we perform 2–4 smaller exercises. On dynamic or max effort day, the hamstrings and lower and upper back must be worked heavily and directly. The abdominals, calves, and connective tissue must be strengthened through a wide range of repetitions of 100 and higher. This is important for storing kinetic energy.

On dynamic day, we do reverse hypers, glute ham raises, or both at a volume of 600 reps per month or 20 reps per day. For reverse hypers, 40–60 reps with heavy weight twice a week works best. That's 240 heavy reverse hypers a week. The total for reverse hyper work is 50 percent of our dynamic day and max effort day.

Lat work is at such a high volume that it's hard to estimate. We work the lats four days a week for more than 300 reps per week. We repeat this week after week.

Abdominal work is also very high volume. When using kettlebells for overall body strength, the repetitions are astronomical.

Sled work for the upper and lower body for strength or strength endurance can take up to two hours of training per week including restoration. All of these movements are performed after the speed or max effort workout. As an alternative to max effort work, the Westside system allows us to alter the work from multijoint training to muscle group isolation as much as possible.

All work is directed to one area. For example, reverse hypers done in a superset fashion will cause massive stimulation in the spinal erector and lumbar region. Performing glute ham raises in supersets of 3–5 reps with ankle weight leg curls in sets of 50 reps will induce a massive amount of blood to the area.

This will increase the number of myofibrils per muscle fiber as well as the filamental area density by increasing the cell size and strength. The side benefit is increased size and strength of the soft tissue, including connective tissue. This will contribute to the ability to control and use a higher amount of kinetic energy. That's how small workouts can increase strength, especially explosive strength.

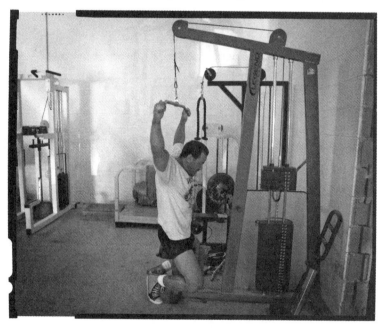

You can also do low back work supersetted with abdominals between the low back sets. A hypertrophy workout for the lower back can be harder to recover from than squatting and deadlifting.

For grip, arms, upper back, and delts, do kettlebell cleans and snatches for 60 seconds of work and 30 seconds of rest between sets or heavy barbell rows for sets of 6–10 reps with kettlebell work.

The workout must be dense, meaning the actual work done in a time period—not including rest—should be intense.

You can't always superset when doing heavy isolated exercises. It depends on your level of preparedness.

Hypertrophy work is always related to fixing a weak muscle group or raising general physical preparedness (GPP) and specialized physical preparation (SPP). See Chapters 17, 21, and 22 for more information.

Here are some hypertrophy exercises listed by muscle group:

Low Back

- Reverse hypers

- Back raises

- 45-degree reverse hypers

- Straight leg deadlifts

- Kettlebell deadlifts

- Kettlebell swings

- Light good mornings

- Band good mornings

Upper Back and Traps

- Kettlebell cleans

- Dumbbell cleans

- Kettlebell snatches

- Barbell power cleans

- Barbell power snatches

- Kettlebell shrugs

- Dumbbell shrugs

- Barbell power shrugs

- Band shrugs

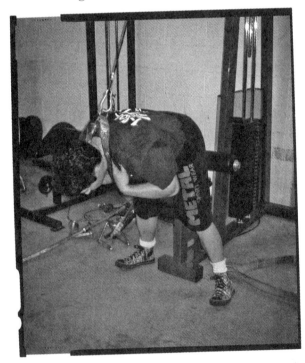

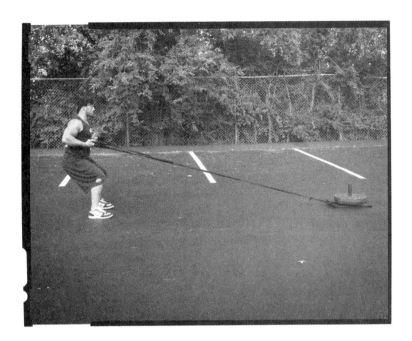

Hamstrings

- Leg curls

- Leg curls on the machine

- Glute ham raises

- Band leg curls

- Reverse hyper leg curls

- Sled pulls

Glutes and Hips

- Sled pulls

- Glute ham raises

All squats, good mornings, and deadlifts will work the hip and glutes. The wider the stance, the more the glutes are worked, and the closer the stance, the more the low back is worked.

Lats

- Barbell rows

- Dumbbell rows

- Kettlebells rows

- Chest-supported rows (Machine lat work will build hypertrophy but not pulling strength.)

- Belt squats

- Squatting with raised heels

- Sled pulls forward, backward, and sideways

- Jumps with weight

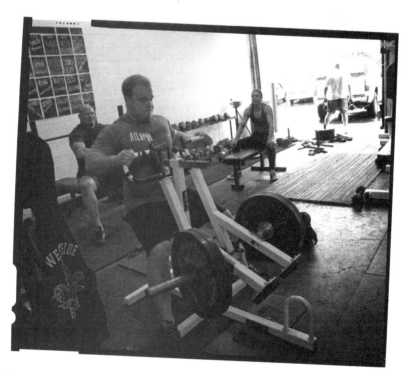

Calves

- Seated calf raises

- Standing calf raises

Rotate individual exercises when the program slows down for each muscle group. There isn't any time schedule, so just do what you need to do, not what you like to do. Choose from very heavy low reps (6–10 reps) to very high reps such as with the ankle weight leg curls, which not only build muscle mass but also thicken the ligaments and tendons. This is very important for preventing injury and increasing the amount of kinetic energy stored in the soft tissue.

And last but not least, squat or deadlift for 1–3 minutes without putting the bar back in the rack for squatting or returning the deadlift to the floor. This will build muscle mass. Squat slowly and eccentrically onto a box or at any speed you like. Hold the movement statically at the top on the box or in any position you like. Use a wide or close stance or change your stance while doing a timed set.

The deadlift can be trained in the same manner.

You will see a substantial increase in your muscularity, and as an added bonus, your grip strength will increase. Bob Peoples trained in this manner years ago, and V. Alexeev, the great Olympic weightlifter, used the same process to gain muscle mass and strength.

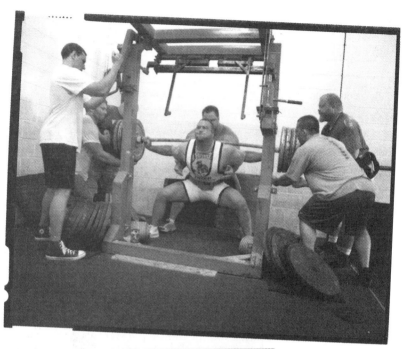

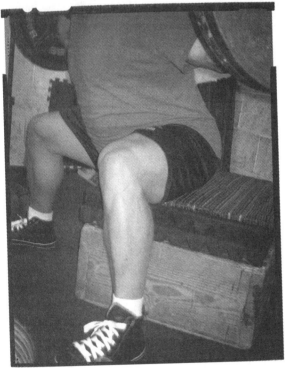

SQUAT TECHNIQUE

Lifters must learn proper squat technique before anything else. The importance of proper technique should be stressed in each and every squat workout. But what is proper squat technique?

Let's start at the feet and work up. The feet or stance should be as wide as possible as long as you can break parallel. This means the feet should be as straight as possible. Larger men and women will have to point their feet out to the sides to some degree to allow them to reach proper depth. You should wear Chuck Taylor's so you can push your feet apart, not down. Pushing the feet apart properly engages the powerful hip muscles. It also allows you to reach depth more easily by shortening the squat stroke. Next, push the knees out to the sides. This forces the hip muscles to engage more powerfully.

The first movement on the descent is to push the hips and glutes backward. Never bend the knees. The shins must remain vertical at all times. By pushing the glutes backward, you are now descending. The stomach must be full of air and pushed in front and out to the sides where the oblique muscles are located. The spinal erectors must be tight and arched. The chest must be full of air with the upper back tight and the shoulder blades pulled together. The chin should be raised because this will tighten up the lats and traps, which is where the bar rests. As you lower into a squat, your eyes should be fixed on something. This will allow you to raise your head slightly on the descent.

To recover from parallel, keep the eyes fixed on the same point as before. To rise from the squat, first push your back into the bar. Remember, this is what we are trying to lift, so push against the bar, not the floor. If you push against the floor, you will tip backward. Then push your knees apart and arch the spinal erectors as much as possible. While continuing to rise, lift the chest and push on the belt as much as possible. You have now recovered from the squat for a three light success.

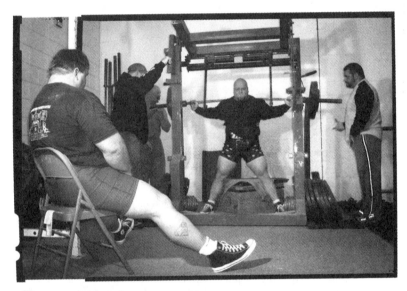

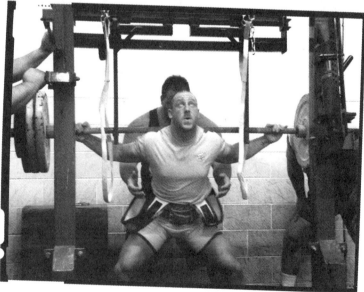

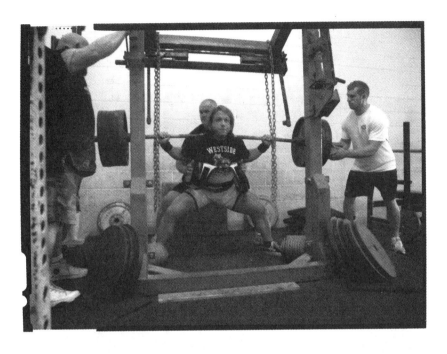

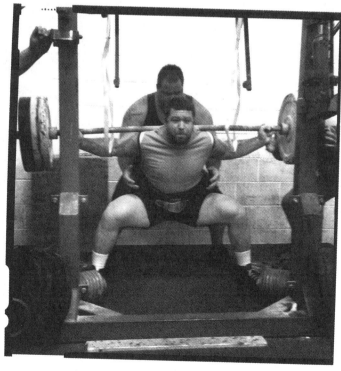

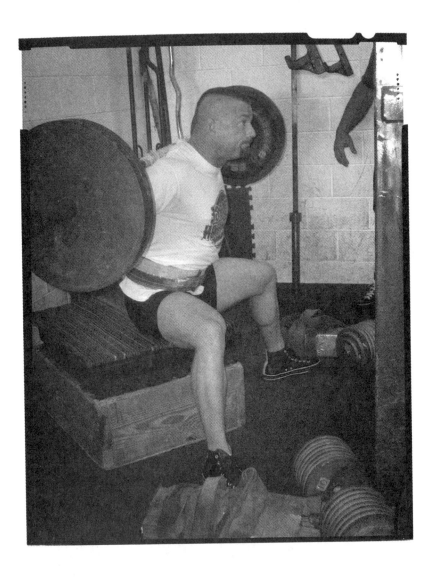

Chapter 12

BOX SQUATTING

Box squatting is simply the most effective method for squatting. It helped produced the first 800-lb squat in 1969, which was done by Pat Casey of the Culver City Westside Barbell Club. Box squatting also helped Pat total the first 2000 lbs and 2100 lbs. In 2008, Vlad Alhazov squatted 1250 lbs for a world record thanks to box squatting in his training.

Mike Bridges said a squat is an arched back good morning at parallel. His squat form was impeccable and was referred to as the "Bridge's flare".

Box squatting involves the same process as a sumo deadlift. There is only one method of box squatting—using a wide stance with the feet pointed as straight forward as possible. Larger lifters will have to point their toes outward somewhat to reach parallel. Push the glutes to the rear by breaking at the hips, not the knees. Push the knees out to the sides during both the eccentric and concentric phases. As with any squat, arch the entire back and raise the chest as you lower yourself onto the box. This keeps the bar placed above the upper thigh at about midpoint. The best squatters lean forward to some extent. The upper thigh should come in contact with the lower abs.

After sitting on the box, relax the hip and glute muscles somewhat to allow yourself to sit or "rock" onto the box. After sitting completely on the box, push against the bar and raise the head to start the concentric phase. If you push with the feet first, you will round over into a good morning. This is caused by the hips rising before the head. Always push the feet apart when squatting on a box in the eccentric phase.

Never push the feet down but rather out to the sides. While on the box, the secret is to have your shins past the point of straight up and down. This will cause you to actually leg curl yourself off the box. All box squats can be at parallel or below all the time. When full squatting, most will squat higher and higher as the weight increases, but by sitting on a predetermined box, all squats are the same depth.

Box squatting is somewhat like proprioceptive neuromuscular facilitation (PNF) stretching, and a squat can be held down for a count of three. While box squatting, one-sixth of your body is suspended off the box, so if you want to build flexibility, you should box squat. To do this, start on a high box of 16 inches. Remove one inch of the mat at a time until you reach the desired depth. You can go from 16 inches to 10 inches in a matter of a few minutes. Each time a mat is removed, push your glutes out to the rear and push your knees apart as much as possible.

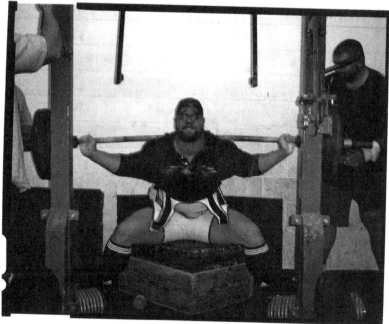

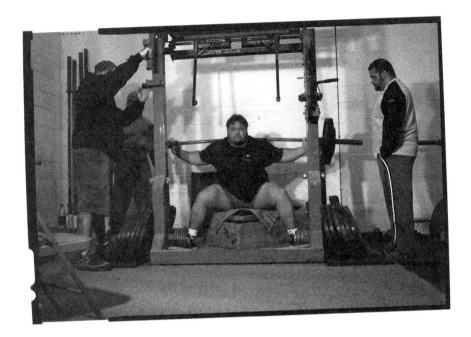

By widening your stance on the same size box, you will increase groin and hip flexibility as well. The increased range of motion comes from a process known as "contract relax antagonist contract", or CRAC (Ethyre-Abraham 1986). All the squat muscles are held static prior to the eccentric phase and relaxed upon contact with the box. Then they contract again to start the concentric phase.

What should your box be made of? The box can be made of wood with rubber mats or if can be made of just wood. It can also be made of foam.

Many feel that box squatting is unsafe. These people don't know the process of proper box squatting. It doesn't cause spinal injuries, and sitting on foam should put most trainers or coaches at rest. By sitting with the shins straight up and down, there isn't any pressure on the patella tendons either. As long as you know how to properly breathe and hold your breath, you'll be fine. The exercise is only as dangerous as the level of ignorance of the trainer. So don't believe what you hear. The box is perfectly safe. Perform the box squat and you'll be on your way to world records just like the young and old have done at Westside.

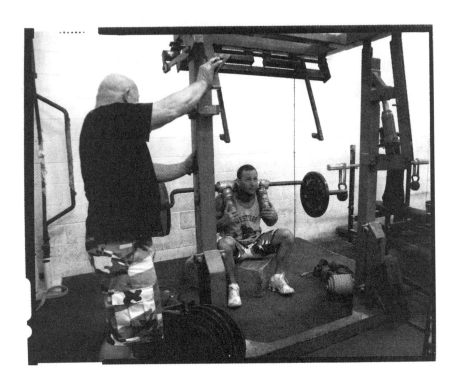

LOADING AND PERIODIZATION

Squat Periodization

Speed-strength, strength-speed, and circa-max waves are done on Fridays. These waves separate the max effort day by three days, which is needed for extreme workouts. Fridays are for multiple sets of two reps and are considered high volume. Bands, which provide overspeed eccentrics, or chains are always used to accommodate resistance. The squats are always done on a hard box or a foam-covered box. Remember, force equals mass times acceleration, which means you can move submaximal weights with maximal speed.

Speed-Strength

Here are some examples of three-week waves for the development of speed-strength. The weight calculations are easy math. As the weight increases, the band tension must increase as well. These waves can be changed into a circa-max phase quite easily.

400-lb squat with a three-week wave:

Week 1: 200 lbs plus 125 lbs band tension for 8 sets of 2 reps
Week 2: 220 lbs plus 125 lbs band tension for 8 sets of 2 reps
Week 3: 240 lbs plus 125 lbs band tension for 6 sets of 2 reps

500-lb squat with a three-week wave:

Week 1: 250 lbs plus 125 lbs band tension for 8 sets of 2 reps
Week 2: 275 lbs plus 125 lbs band tension for 8 sets of 2 reps
Week 3: 300 lbs plus 125 lbs band tension for 6 sets of 2 reps

600-squat with a three-week wave:

Week 1: 300 lbs plus 150 lbs band tension for 8 sets of 2 reps
Week 2: 330 lbs plus 150 lbs band tension for 8 sets of 2 reps
Week 3: 360 lbs plus 150 lbs band tension for 6 sets of 2 reps

800-lb squat with a three-week wave:

Week 1: 400 lbs plus 200 lbs band tension for 8 sets of 2 reps
Week 2: 440 lbs plus 200 lbs band tension for 8 sets of 2 reps
Week 3: 480 lbs plus 200 lbs band tension for 8 sets of 2 reps

Circa-Max

You must be in shape and able to break a box squat record in order to start a two-week circa-max phase. If these two factors are in place, you should be able to accomplish a contest record. The waves are reduced to one-week waves due to the demands that large amounts of band tension can place on the body. Three-week waves with bands can cause a negative effect on the deadlift because of the prolonged fatigue effect.

Here are some examples of circa-max phase training. The sets with added band tension are at 90–97 percent. The virtual force effect is much greater than one can imagine.

800-lb max

Week 1: 375 lbs at the top with bands

- Warm up

- 315 lbs x 2 reps

- 365 lbs x 2 reps

- 415 lbs x 2 reps

- 440 lbs x 1 rep

- 465 lbs x 1 rep

Week 2: Warm up

- 315 lbs x 2 reps

- 370 lbs x 2 reps

- 415 lbs x 1 rep

- 465 lbs x 1 rep

- 515 lbs x 1 rep personal record

Week 3: Warm up and reduce the band tension to 250 lbs at the top

- 315 lbs x 2 reps

- 370 lbs x 1 rep

- 415 lbs x 1 rep

Week 4: 500 lbs with 375 lbs of band tension (This will produce a 800-lb meet squat.)

To squat 800 lbs or more, you must add weight to the max done in the second week. If you box squat 550 lbs or more, the 375 lbs of band tension should give you a contest squat of 850 lbs. There are five Westside squatters who have done 900 lbs after doing 600 lbs of bar weight with 375 lbs of band tension. With the barbell representing 66 percent of a contest squat, this should hold true with a variable of six percent up or down. "Dollar Bill" is six feet, one inch with a body weight of 308 lbs. He made his first 905-lb squat after doing 600 lbs plus 375 lbs of band tension. Phil Harrington is five feet, eight inches and 181 lbs. He made a 905-lb world record side by side with Dollar Bill.

Here is their circa-max phase:

Week 1: 405 lbs x 2 reps plus 375 lbs band tension

- 475 lbs x 2 reps plus 375 lbs band tension

- 530 lbs x 2 reps plus 375 lbs band tension

- 565 lbs x 1 rep plus 375 lbs band tension

Week 2: 405 lbs x 2 reps plus 375 lbs band tension

- 475 lbs x 2 reps plus 375 lbs band tension

- 530 lbs x 1 rep plus 375 lbs band tension

- 570 lbs x 1 rep plus 375 lbs band tension

- 600 lbs x 1 rep plus 375 lbs band tension (PR)

The circa-max workout is on Fridays. In order to do the circa-max work, you must be physically and psychologically prepared. If you're prepared to do a new box squat record, you should be able to break a new meet squat record. You must wear your meet gear with the straps down, but don't wear knee wraps.

You must duplicate the eccentric time phase at a meet while on the box. This will keep your timing on track. If your box squat eccentric is 0.51 second and it takes you 2.5 seconds to reach parallel at a contest, your reversal timing will be off.

Circa-Max for 1000-lb Squat

For a 1000-lb squat, you must raise the band tension to roughly 440 lbs at the top. For a 1000-lb contest squat, a box squat of 600 lbs of bar weight plus the 440 lbs of band tension must be accomplished at parallel. The lifters at Westside who have progressed from 900 lbs have followed this system. As the bar weight grows to about 650 lbs, the contest squat moves to 1050 lbs. Panora, Wenning, and Bolognone experienced this progression. The lifters who can move these weights the fastest will have the largest carryover from the box squat to an actual contest squat.

Here's an example of a two-week wave for the circa-max phase for a 1000-lb squat:

Week 1: 475 lbs x 2 reps plus 440 lbs band tension

- 525 lbs x 2 reps plus 440 lbs band tension

- 550 lbs x 1 rep plus 440 lbs band tension

- 575 lbs x 1 rep plus 440 lbs band tension

Week 2: Warm up

- 455 lbs x 2 reps plus band tension

- 525 lbs x 2 reps plus band tension

- 560 lbs x 1 rep plus band tension

- 580 lbs x 1 rep plus band tension

- 605 lbs x 1 rep plus band tension (PR)

Week 3: Download for delayed training effect. This is essential for the body to recover and for hormonal activities to increase (Nazny, 1983).

As you go from an 800-lb squat to a 900-lb squat to a 1000-lb squat, the bar weight is raised by 100 lbs in order for you to advance from 800 lbs to 900 lbs. To raise the squat to 1000 lbs, the band tension goes from 375 lbs to 440 lbs. As the squat grows, this requires combination changes of at least 60 percent bar weight up to 66 percent band tension.

The heavy two-week wave is to secure a deadlift at the meet. Experiments with three- or four-week circa-max waves led to overtraining. The distribution of squats on Fridays and max effort work on Mondays must be alternated drastically because the normal loading of squatting on Fridays is 48–80 lifts when training with loads of 75–85 percent per month. Now the average load is 90–97 percent. So the lifts on Mondays, or max effort day, must be removed and replaced with more moderate loads of reverse hypers, glute ham raises, and back raises. These movements should become the main workouts for the two-week wave.

Multi-Week Waves

Westside doesn't recommend that lifters use a special bar on squat day for any length of time. Chuck Vogelpohl said it would distort squat form. I totally agree with this because the special bar will alter your form and use the squatting muscles in a different way. If you must, use something like a Safety squat bar.

Here's a nine-week preparatory cycle, or pendulum wave, that will take you from the early stages of training to an 800–850-lb squat in nine weeks of training:

Week 1: 345 lbs plus 70 lbs band tension for 8 sets x 2 reps

Week 2: 395 lbs plus 70 lbs band tension for 8 sets x 2 reps

Week 3: 435 lbs plus 70 lbs band tension for 6 sets x 2 reps

Week 4: 345 lbs plus 140 lbs band tension for 8 sets x 2 reps

Week 5: 395 lbs plus 140 lbs band tension for 8 sets x 2 reps

Week 6: 435 lbs plus 140 lbs band tension for 6 sets x 2 reps

Week 7: 345 lbs plus 220 lbs band tension for 8 sets x 2 reps

Week 8: 395 lbs plus 220 lbs band tension for 8 sets x 2 reps

Week 9: 435 lbs plus 220 lbs band tension for 6 sets x 2 reps

The ocean is made up of countless waves that are large and small and so is strength training. After three weeks, we could find that we aren't any stronger or faster. V. Alexeev, the great Olympic champion, found this to be true for himself. This was told to me by the late Mel Siff, PhD.

Three-week waves are most common in training. When using an enormous amount of band tension equal to or above the amount of bar weight, the wave must be shortened to two weeks (i.e. strength-speed). The band tension can cause extreme stress on the muscular and connective tissues. Remember, max effort day is rotated each week. There isn't any gradual wave here.

As you can see, squat training is mostly three-week waves. For a powerlifter, it looks like 50 percent up to 60 percent. These percentages represent a squat with contest gear, knee wraps, and the straps up. The box squats are done with the straps down and without knee wraps. For sportsmen who do not squat in power meets, the box squats represent 75–85 percent of a one rep max on the box squat.

After squatting on Friday, speed pulls are done 80 percent of the time with bar weight and band tension of 220 lbs at the top. This works fine for lifters who deadlift 800 lbs or less. Lifters who pull more than 800 lbs should use 280 lbs of band tension in addition to the bar weight. Rack pulls can be done after squatting. Always train your lower back, hamstrings, and abs after squatting. These are examples of how to wave from strength-speed to speed-strength to circa-max waves.

Dynamic Method

The dynamic method is used to build a fast rate of force development and explosive strength. Multiple sets are used, and half of the time the weight is at 75–85 percent of a one rep max. Westside uses sets of two reps for up to 12 sets with weights in the 70 percent range. At 80 percent, the total lifts are held to a limit of 10 sets of two reps. The bar speed shouldn't be any lower than one meter per second (m/s) or force production will diminish. For more information, refer to Hill's equation for muscle contraction in Supertraining.

When using the dynamic effort method, always use some form of accommodating resistance. If you are in great shape, your level of physical preparedness will allow you to limit your contest cycle to three weeks—two for the circa-max phase and one deload week. Johnny Parker, the renowned NFL strength coach with four Super Bowl rings, relayed a story about a former Soviet strength coach he had a conversation with years ago.

Johnny asked the coach what to do for his players after a game on Monday. The Soviet coach said, "Work their legs." Johnny said, "What about on Tuesday?" The coach replied again with "work their legs." Johnny asked what to do for Wednesday, and once again, the Soviet coach said, "Work their legs." Johnny asked him what he meant. The former Soviet coach said, "Just change the exercises." This is the conjugate system—constantly switch the exercises. Ben Tabachnic, PhD, said that to adapt to training is to never adapt to training.

Lactic Acid Tolerance Training

Performing up to 20 sets of squats or deadlifts can produce a large amount of lactic acid buildup in the body. This causes the production of growth hormones, which builds muscle mass and raises the anaerobe threshold. The rest periods must be short, about 30–40 seconds. A manageable weight must be utilized, and the bar speed must remain constant throughout the sets. This system works well for not only Olympic lifters or powerlifters but also ball players. The lifter's form must not deteriorate, and the rest periods can't be prolonged in order to recover from large training loads. With high or low intensities, the lifter must be in good shape for his sport. A swimmer must train to swim, a runner must train to run great distances or short sprinting, and a lifter must train for heavy lifting.

Squat Loading

The cornerstone of training is to load by volume and intensity zone. Lifters must adhere to a specified number of barbell lifts per workout at a certain percentage in order to be successful when using chains and weight for squatting. A powerlifter using gear should be at 50–60 percent of a one rep max. Twenty-four lifts is the maximum number of lifts per workout. Twelve lifts is the minimum and 18 is the optimal number.

Let's look at several examples for squatting 600, 800, and 900 lbs using a three-week wave with a 7–14 day delayed transformation leading into the contest.

Example #1: 600-lb squat with a volume of 7200 lbs

300 lbs	120 lbs chains	12 sets of 2 reps	50%
330 lbs	120 lbs chains	12 sets of 2 reps	55%
360 lbs	120 lbs chains	10 sets of 2 reps	60%

Use maximum speed on each rep (force equals mass times acceleration). The volume is essential. By calculating the total lifts per workout, it takes 7200 lbs to accomplish or maintain a 600-lb squat.

Example #2: 800-lb max with a volume of 9600 lbs

405 lbs	160 lbs chains	12 sets of 2 reps	50%
440 lbs	160 lbs chains	12 sets of 2 reps	55%
480 lbs	120 lbs chains	10 sets of 2 reps	60%

Use the same delayed transformation period. To squat 800 lbs or maintain that strength, you must maintain 9600 lbs of volume.

Example #3: 900-lb squat max with a volume of 10,800 lbs

450 lbs	200 lbs chains	12 sets of 2 reps	50%
500 lbs	200 lbs chains	12 sets of 2 reps	55%
540 lbs	200 lbs chains	10 sets of 2 reps	60%

Use the same math and total number of lifts and you won't over- or under-train for a record attempt. The chains provide accommodating resistance but shouldn't be added as bar weight. I've listed the most successful amount of chains to use according to your maximal squat strength

Using Bands Plus Weight for the Squat

You must be precise with the amount of band tension and weight because if you have too much you will fail. To squat 800 lbs, a max single would require 500 lbs of bar weight plus 375 lbs of band tension. A 900-lb squat would require 600 lbs of bar weight and 375 lbs of band tension. A 1000-lb squat would require 600 lbs of bar weight and 440 lbs of band tension. Note the increased band tension.

Very technical squatters can and have squatted the top end volume. For example, Tony Ramos and Mark Burrows made their first 800-lb squats in a meet with 500 lbs plus 375 lbs of band tension (a strong and medium band). Make sure you weigh your band tension. Mark made a 925-lb squat with 600 lbs of bar weight and 375 lbs of band tension. I made a 920-lb squat at a meet with a box squat of 600 lbs plus 375 lbs of band tension. Presently at Westside, we have 14 men who squat over 1000 lbs and four over 1100 lbs.

Tony Bolognone made a 1000-lb squat with 600 lbs of bar weight and 440 lbs of band tension. He also made a 1025-lb squat with 620 lbs of bar weight plus 440 lbs of band tension. Tony has progressed to 1075 lbs and an 1100-lb max squat in a meet. The bar weight was 700 lbs, and the band tension was 440 lbs. The progress that Tony has made squatting at a meet mirrors his gains on the box squat with bar weight plus band tension.

Bar loading with band tension is somewhat different from chain loading. Why? Bands provide overspeed eccentrics that can cause severe soreness in the early stages of training. They also provide accommodating resistance, which provides near maximum force throughout the entire range of motion. The total number of lifts with small amounts of band tension will be close to chain loading. However, when a circa-max cycle lasting two weeks is used, the band tension is around 40–45 percent. Pure strength-speed work requires 50 percent or more total resistance, which is provided by band tension.

A circa-max contest phase should look like this:

Example #1: 800-lb max squat during week one

400 lbs	2 rep	375 lbs band tension
425 lbs	2 rep	375 lbs band tension
450 lbs	2 rep	375 lbs band tension
475 lbs	1 rep	375 lbs band tension

Westside recommends seven total lifts at 90 percent or more and 4–10 lifts.

Example #2: 800-lb max squat during week two

400 lbs	2 rep	375 lbs band tension
440 lbs	2 rep	375 lbs band tension
475 lbs	1 rep	375 lbs band tension
500 lbs	1 rep	375 lbs band tension

If you fail at a meet, your box height is incorrect or your form isn't good. Note: You must use perfect form with every rep whether you're using light or heavy weight. A deloading week is required to recover from the immense work load.

For week three, warm up and do three sets of two reps with 405 lbs and 140 lbs of band tension. Always continue the special exercises.

Example #1: 900-lb squat

Week 1		
405 lbs	2 rep	375 lbs band tension
475 lbs	2 rep	375 lbs band tension
520 lbs	1 rep	375 lbs band tension
575 lbs	1 rep	375 lbs band tension

Week 2		
405 lbs	2 rep	375 lbs band tension
475 lbs	2 rep	375 lbs band tension
520 lbs	1 rep	375 lbs band tension
570 lbs	1 rep	375 lbs band tension

Week 3:

Again, deloading must occur to receive the full benefits of the circa-max two-week wave. For the deload week, warm up and perform three sets of two reps with 500 lbs of bar weight and 140 lbs of band tension.

Example #2: 1000-lb max squat

Week 1 (after the warm up)		
475 lbs	2 rep	440 lbs band tension
500 lbs	2 rep	440 lbs band tension
540 lbs	2 rep	440 lbs band tension
575 lbs	1 rep	440 lbs band tension

Week 2 (after the warm up)		
475 lbs	2 rep	440 lbs band tension
520 lbs	2 rep	440 lbs band tension
540 lbs	2 rep	440 lbs band tension
570 lbs	1 rep	440 lbs band tension
600 lbs	1 rep	440 lbs band tension

Week 3:

Deload to provide delayed transformation. Do 550 lbs for two reps with 250 lbs of band tension. Don't neglect the special exercises. The circa-max phase should last two weeks with one week for deloading leading into a meet.

In the late 1990s and early 2000s, we used a three-week circa-max wave. It was done doing five sets of two reps. The total weight (band tension and bar weight at the top) was above 90 percent and up to slightly above 100 percent. I used the same 485 lbs plus 375 lbs of band tension at the top. This is equal to 860 lbs. I squatted 805 lbs up to 920 lbs. I estimate I had 50 lbs to spare. This was good for the squat but not for the deadlift. As our squats continued to go up, the deadlifts stalled. At that time (about ten years ago), we took a top weight band squat at any time we desired. We reduced the circa-max to two weeks and the squats still made progress, but now the deadlifts started going up again. We started intensifying our deadlift volume on speed squat day (Fridays), and on

Mondays, we started deadlifting more. The theory was that we weren't conditioned to deadlift.

Deadlift Loading

On max effort day for the squat and deadlift, we use three primary exercises. We do a special squat or special deadlift or a form of good mornings for maxing out. We never use a regular contest style squat on max effort day. A regular deadlift is seldom done except for maybe twice a year at most. The lifts on max effort day should be scheduled like meets—three lifts at 90 percent and up for a new max. After warming up to 90 percent for one rep, we do a second single at close to a new gym record and then a third single for a small personal record. Westside has kept records for the past 25 years because we've used this loading system. You must strive to raise your top limit by a small margin. Switch each week to different core exercises, and only perform good mornings for a three or five rep max. Follow up with 2–4 small exercises.

After squatting on speed squat day or sometimes before, we choose a deadlift program. We perform it in a rack for a three-week wave using band tension of three different strengths—125 lbs of mini-bands quadrupled, 250 lbs of monster mini-bands quadrupled, or 325 lbs of light bands quadrupled. As the squat workout intensity increases, the deadlift work is in a reverse wave. In other words, most three-week waves begin with the easiest work load first. However, the three-week wave for the deadlift begins with the most intense set first.

For example:

Week 1	315 lbs	10 × 2 reps	350 lbs band tension
Week 2	315 lbs	8 × 2 reps	250 lbs band tension
Week 3	225 lbs	8 × 3 reps	250 lbs band tension

The deadlifts are performed conventional style without any straps in a power rack off a pin setting that places the plates five to seven inches off the floor. The example above is based on a 700-lb deadlifter. An 800-lb deadlifter would use an additional 90 lbs of bar weight. This style of band deadlifts will greatly increase the squat as well as the deadlift. It's a substitute for the high-rep Dimel deadlifts, which are performed four times a week.

Use about 25–35 percent of your one rep max on the deadlift and do two sets of 20 reps. If this is out of your physical preparedness level, do four sets of ten reps. This system of deadlifting adds muscle mass and shouldn't be performed for more than 14 days, which equals eight workouts, or the training effect will decrease. This type of training raised Matt Dimel from a stalled 820-lb squat for one year to a 1010-lb squat in 13 months, which was the world record in the super heavyweight division at the time. Steve Wilson was training with Matt during the same time, and he increased his stalled deadlift of 810 lbs to 865 lbs at a body weight of 265 lbs in the same 13 months.

Speed pulls off the floor are another variety of deadlifting after speed squatting. Use band tension of 100 lbs at floor level and 220 lbs at lockout. At 57 years old, I made 715 lbs at a body weight of 217 lbs using this method. I used speed pulls of 345 lbs of bar weight plus 220 lbs of band tension added at lockout for single reps and 8–12 lifts done ultra-wide sumo style. The best single in this style was 535 lbs. An 800-lb deadlifter would use 280 lbs of band tension at lockout. A 585-lb single using the ultra-wide sumo style has produced three 800-lb deadlifters—two sumo style and one conventional style. Remember, the speed day volume must be high with an intensity of 50–85 percent. The max effort day must be reversed and have a maximum intensity of roughly 50 percent of the volume to form a wave between volume and intensity zones.

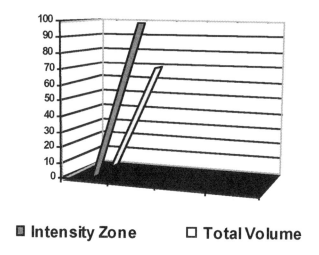

Squat and Deadlift Max Effort Day

■ **Intensity Zone**   □ **Total Volume**

Figure 1: Low volume training; highest intensity possible for 100 percent and above; limit to three lifts of 90 percent and above.

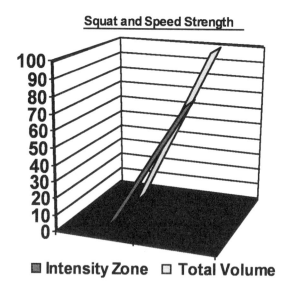

Squat and Speed Strength

■ **Intensity Zone** □ **Total Volume**

Figure 2: High volume training; moderate intensity zones between 60–85 percent; limit to 12–24 lifts per training session.

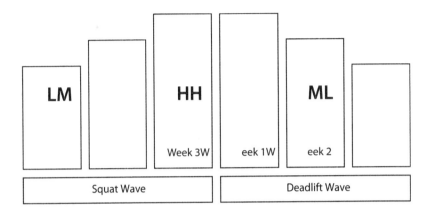

Figure 3: Combining squatting and deadlifting speed work.

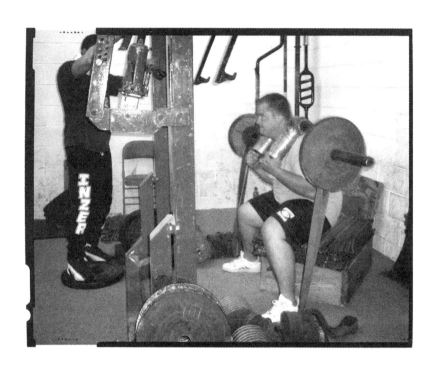

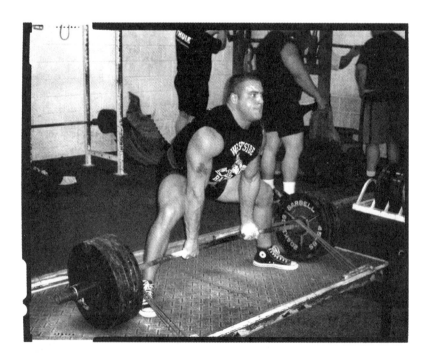

Chapter 14

SAMPLE SPEED WORKOUTS

Because we use a three-week pendulum wave, I will outline a series of three, three-week waves that our top squatters use and rotate every three weeks.

1. A. J. Roberts, 1008 lbs at a body weight of 308 lbs, uses a Mastodon squat bar plus bands on a box below parallel for his speed-strength cycle.

Week 1	500 lbs bar weight	140 lbs band tension	8 sets, 2 reps
Week 2	550 lbs bar weight	140 lbs band tension	8 sets, 2 reps
Week 3	600 lbs bar weight	140 lbs band tension	6 sets, 2 reps
Week 4	500 lbs bar weight	250 lbs band tension	8 sets, 2 reps
Week 5	550 lbs bar weight	250 lbs band tension	8 sets, 2 reps
Week 6	600 lbs bar weight	250 lbs band tension	6 sets, 2 reps
Week 7	500 lbs bar weight	375 lbs band tension	8 sets, 2 reps
Week 8	550 lbs bar weight	375 lbs band tension	8 sets, 2 reps
Week 9	600 lbs bar weight	375 lbs band tension	6 sets, 2 reps

2. Matt Smith, 1160 lbs as a super heavyweight, uses a 14-inch cambered bar on a box below parallel for his speed-strength cycle.

Week 1	580 lbs bar weight	160 lbs chains	8 sets, 2 reps
Week 2	580 lbs bar weight	160 lbs chains	8 sets, 2 reps
Week 3	580 lbs bar weight	160 lbs chains	6 sets, 2 reps
Week 4	640 lbs bar weight	240 lbs chains	8 sets, 2 reps
Week 5	640 lbs bar weight	240 lbs chains	8 sets, 2 reps
Week 6	640 lbs bar weight	240 lbs chains	6 sets, 2 reps
Week 7	690 lbs bar weight	320 lbs chains	8 sets, 2 reps
Week 8	690 lbs bar weight	320 lbs chains	8 sets, 2 reps
Week 9	690 lbs bar weight	320 lbs chains	6 sets, 2 reps

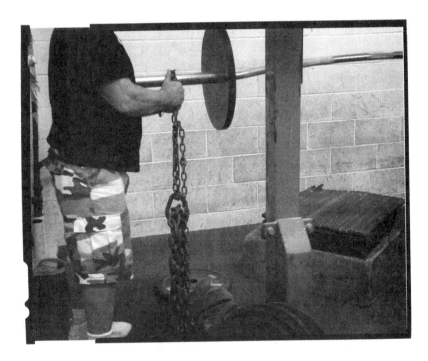

3. Vlad Alhazov, 1155 lbs as a super heavyweight, uses a bow bar with a two-inch cambered bar done on a box below parallel.

Week 1	500 lbs bar weight	140 lbs band tension	8 sets, 2 reps
Week 2	550 lbs bar weight	140 lbs band tension	8 sets, 2 reps
Week 3	600 lbs bar weight	140 lbs band tension	6 sets, 2 reps
Week 4	500 lbs bar weight	250 lbs band tension	8 sets, 2 reps
Week 5	550 lbs bar weight	250 lbs band tension	8 sets, 2 reps
Week 6	600 lbs bar weight	250 lbs band tension	6 sets, 2 reps
Week 7	500 lbs bar weight	375 lbs band tension	8 sets, 2 reps
Week 8	550 lbs bar weight	375 lbs band tension	8 sets, 2 reps
Week 9	600 lbs bar weight	375 lbs band tension	6 sets, 2 reps

4. Tony Bolognone, a 1075-lb squatter as a super heavyweight, uses a Safety squat bar and a close stance with explosive power on a box below parallel. His strength-speed cycle is for two weeks on a box below parallel.

Week 1	350 lbs bar weight	140 lbs weight releasers	8 sets, 2 reps
Week 2	420 lbs bar weight	140 lbs weight releasers	8 sets, 2 reps
Week 3	490 lbs bar weight	140 lbs weight releasers	6 sets, 2 reps
Week 4	350 lbs bar weight	140 lbs weight releasers	8 sets, 2 reps
Week 5	420 lbs bar weight	140 lbs weight releasers	8 sets, 2 reps
Week 6	490 lbs bar weight	140 lbs weight releasers	6 sets, 2 reps
Week 7	350 lbs bar weight	140 lbs weight releasers	8 sets, 2 reps
Week 8	420 lbs bar weight	140 lbs weight releasers	8 sets, 2 reps
Week 9	490 lbs bar weight	140 lbs weight releasers	6 sets, 2 reps

5. Greg Panora, who is a 1060-lb squatter at a body weight of 242 lbs, uses a Mastodon bar. His strength-speed cycle is for two weeks on a box below parallel.

Week 1	500 lbs bar weight	500 lbs band tension	1 set, 2 reps
Week 1	500 lbs bar weight	500 lbs band tension	1 set, 2 reps
Week 1	550 lbs bar weight	500 lbs band tension	1 set, 2 reps
Week 2	550 lbs bar weight	500 lbs band tension	1 set, 2 reps
Week 2	575 lbs bar weight	500 lbs band tension	1 set, 2 reps
Week 2	600 lbs bar weight	500 lbs band tension	1 set, 2 reps

6. Luke Edwards, 1015 lbs at a body weight of 275 lbs, uses a Mastodon bar on a box below parallel for his two-week strength-speed cycle.

Week 1	500 lbs bar weight	500 lbs band tension	1 set, 2 reps
Week 1	500 lbs bar weight	500 lbs band tension	1 set, 2 reps
Week 1	525 lbs bar weight	500 lbs band tension	1 set, 2 reps
Week 2	500 lbs bar weight	500 lbs band tension	1 set, 2 reps
Week 2	550 lbs bar weight	500 lbs band tension	1 set, 2 reps
Week 2	575 lbs bar weight	500 lbs band tension	1 set, 1 reps

7. Dave Hoff is a 1005-lb squatter at a body weight of 275 lbs. This is a circa-max phase cycle.

Week 1	500 lbs bar weight	440 lbs band tension	1 set, 2 reps
Week 1	500 lbs bar weight	440 lbs band tension	1 set, 2 reps
Week 1	540 lbs bar weight	440 lbs band tension	1 set, 2 reps
Week 1	575 lbs bar weight	440 lbs band tension	1 set, 1 reps
Week 2	500 lbs bar weight	440 lbs band tension	1 set, 2 reps
Week 2	540 lbs bar weight	440 lbs band tension	1 set, 2 reps
Week 2	580 lbs bar weight	440 lbs band tension	1 set, 1 reps
Week 2	605 lbs bar weight	440 lbs band tension	1 set, 1 reps

This is delayed transformation on a box below parallel.

Week 3	500 lbs bar weight	250 lbs band tension	1 set, 2 reps
Week 3	500 lbs bar weight	250 lbs band tension	1 set, 2 reps
Week 3	500 lbs bar weight	250 lbs band tension	1 set, 2 reps

8. Phil Harrington is a 905-lb squatter at a body weight of 181 lbs. This is a two-week circa-max phase cycle on a box below parallel as well as a deload week or delayed transformation.

Week 1	470 lbs bar weight	375 lbs band tension	1 set, 2 reps
Week 1	520 lbs bar weight	375 lbs band tension	1 set, 2 reps
Week 1	550 lbs bar weight	375 lbs band tension	1 set, 2 reps
Week 1	575 lbs bar weight	375 lbs band tension	1 set, 1 reps
Week 2	470 lbs bar weight	375 lbs band tension	1 set, 2 reps
Week 2	520 lbs bar weight	375 lbs band tension	1 set, 2 reps
Week 2	550 lbs bar weight	375 lbs band tension	1 set, 1 reps
Week 2	580 lbs bar weight	375 lbs band tension	1 set, 1 reps
Week 3	605 lbs bar weight	375 lbs band tension	1 set, 1 reps
Week 3	470 lbs bar weight	140 lbs band tension	1 set, 2 reps
Week 3	470 lbs bar weight	140 lbs band tension	1 set, 2 reps
Week 3	470 lbs bar weight	140 lbs band tension	1 set, 2 reps

9. Louie Simmons is a 920-lb squatter at a body weight of 242 lbs with a front squat speed-strength cycle on a box below parallel.

Week 1	250 lbs bar weight	70 lbs band tension	8 sets, 3 reps
Week 2	275 lbs bar weight	70 lbs band tension	8 sets, 2 reps
Week 3	300 lbs bar weight	70 lbs band tension	6 sets, 2 reps
Week 4	250 lbs bar weight	140 lbs band tension	8 sets, 3 reps
Week 5	275 lbs bar weight	140 lbs band tension	8 sets, 3 reps
Week 6	300 lbs bar weight	140 lbs band tension	6 sets, 2 reps
Week 7	250 lbs bar weight	250 lbs band tension	8 sets, 3 reps
Week 8	275 lbs bar weight	250 lbs band tension	8 sets, 3 reps
Week 9	300 lbs bar weight	250 lbs band tension	6 sets, 2 reps

10. Tony Ramos is an 810-lb squatter at a body weight of 181 lbs on a strength-speed cycle on a box below parallel.

Week 1	405 lbs bar weight	120 lbs chains	10 sets, 2 reps
Week 2	440 lbs bar weight	120 lbs chains	10 sets, 2 reps
Week 3	480 lbs bar weight	120 lbs chains	8 sets, 2 reps
Week 4	405 lbs bar weight	160 lbs chains	10 sets, 2 reps
Week 5	440 lbs bar weight	160 lbs chains	10 sets, 2 reps
Week 6	480 lbs bar weight	160 lbs chains	8 sets, 2 reps
Week 7	405 lbs bar weight	200 lbs chains	10 sets, 2 reps
Week 8	440 lbs bar weight	200 lbs chains	10 sets, 2 reps
Week 9	480 lbs bar weight	200 lbs chains	8 sets, 2 reps

11. Dave Cook is a 700-lb squatter on a strength-speed cycle on a box below parallel.

Week 1	350 lbs bar weight	80 lbs chains	10 sets, 2 reps
Week 2	385 lbs bar weight	80 lbs chains	10 sets, 2 reps
Week 3	420 lbs bar weight	80 lbs chains	8 sets, 2 reps
Week 4	350 lbs bar weight	120 lbs chains	10 sets, 2 reps
Week 5	385 lbs bar weight	120 lbs chains	10 sets, 2 reps
Week 6	420 lbs bar weight	120 lbs chains	8 sets, 2 reps
Week 7	350 lbs bar weight	160 lbs chains	10 sets, 2 reps
Week 8	385 lbs bar weight	160 lbs chains	10 sets, 2 reps
Week 9	420 lbs bar weight	160 lbs chains	8 sets, 2 reps

12. Shawn Nutter is a 900-lb squatter doing a circa-max phase on a box below parallel.

Week 1	420 lbs bar weight	375 lbs band tension	1 set, 2 reps
Week 1	470 lbs bar weight	375 lbs band tension	1 set, 2 reps
Week 1	520 lbs bar weight	375 lbs band tension	1 set, 2 reps
Week 1	565 lbs bar weight	375 lbs band tension	1 set, 1 reps
Week 2	420 lbs bar weight	375 lbs band tension	1 set, 2 reps
Week 2	470 lbs bar weight	375 lbs band tension	1 set, 2 reps
Week 2	520 lbs bar weight	375 lbs band tension	1 set, 1 reps
Week 2	570 lbs bar weight	375 lbs band tension	1 set, 1 reps
Week 2	610 lbs bar weight	375 lbs band tension	1 set, 1 reps for PR
Week 3	405 lbs bar weight	140 lbs band tension	1 set, 2 reps
Week 3	405 lbs bar weight	140 lbs band tension	1 set, 2 reps

13. Tony Ramos is at a body weight of 181 lbs doing a circa-max phase at 810 lbs on a box below parallel.

Week 1	385 lbs bar weight	375 lbs band tension	1 set, 2 reps
Week 1	420 lbs bar weight	375 lbs band tension	1 set, 2 reps
Week 1	450 lbs bar weight	375 lbs band tension	1 set, 2 reps
Week 1	470 lbs bar weight	375 lbs band tension	1 set, 1 rep
Week 2	420 lbs bar weight	375 lbs band tension	1 set, 2 reps
Week 2	475 lbs bar weight	375 lbs band tension	1 set, 1 rep
Week 2	520 lbs bar weight	375 lbs band tension	1 set, 1 rep for PR
Week 3	405 lbs bar weight	70 lbs band tension	1 set, 2 reps
Week 3	405 lbs bar weight	70 lbs band tension	1 set, 2 reps
Week 3	405 lbs bar weight	70 lbs band tension	1 set, 2 reps

14. Tony Bolognone is a 1100-lb squatter using a speed-strength wave on a box below parallel.

Week 1	550 lbs bar weight	250 lbs band tension	10 sets, 2 reps
Week 2	610 lbs bar weight	250 lbs band tension	10 sets, 2 reps
Week 3	660 lbs bar weight	250 lbs band tension	10 sets, 2 reps
Week 4	550 lbs bar weight	250 lbs band tension	10 sets, 2 reps
Week 5	610 lbs bar weight	250 lbs band tension	10 sets, 2 reps
Week 6	660 lbs bar weight	250 lbs band tension	10 sets, 2 reps
Week 7	550 lbs bar weight	250 lbs band tension	10 sets, 2 reps
Week 8	610 lbs bar weight	250 lbs band tension	10 sets, 2 reps
Week 9	660 lbs bar weight	250 lbs band tension	10 sets, 2 reps

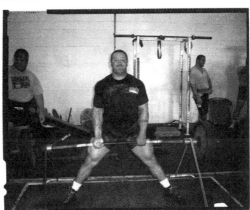

Shaun Nutter

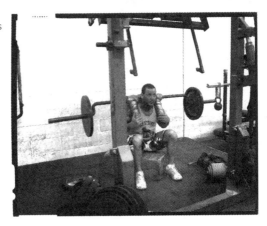

Tony Ramos

15. Amy Weisberger is a 590-lb squatter using a strength-speed wave on a box below parallel.

Week 1	300 lbs bar weight	70 lbs band tension	8 sets, 2 reps
Week 2	330 lbs bar weight	70 lbs band tension	8 sets, 2 reps
Week 3	360 lbs bar weight	70 lbs band tension	8 sets, 2 reps
Week 4	300 lbs bar weight	70 lbs band tension	8 sets, 2 reps
Week 5	330 lbs bar weight	70 lbs band tension	8 sets, 2 reps
Week 6	360 lbs bar weight	70 lbs band tension	8 sets, 2 reps

The second wave is strength-speed.

Week 1	300 lbs bar weight	340 lbs band tension	3 sets, 2 reps
Week 2	330 lbs bar weight	340 lbs band tension	3 sets, 2 reps

The third wave is the reactive method on a box below parallel.

Week 1	300 lbs bar weight	120 lbs weight releasers	10 sets, 2 reps
Week 2	330 lbs bar weight	120 lbs weight releasers	10 sets, 2 reps
Week 3	360 lbs bar weight	120 lbs weight releasers	8 sets, 2 reps

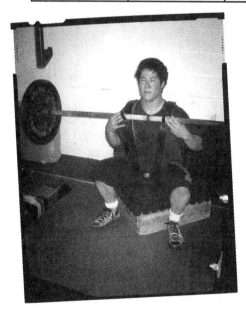

16. Laura Phelps is a 770-lb squatter at a body weight of 181 lbs using a speed-strength wave on a box below parallel.

Week 1	385 lbs bar weight	200 lbs band tension	8 sets, 2 reps
Week 2	425 lbs bar weight	200 lbs band tension	8 sets, 2 reps
Week 3	460 lbs bar weight	200 lbs band tension	8 sets, 2 reps
Week 4	385 lbs bar weight	200 lbs band tension	8 sets, 2 reps
Week 5	425 lbs bar weight	200 lbs band tension	8 sets, 2 reps
Week 6	460 lbs bar weight	200 lbs band tension	6 sets, 2 reps

This is her strength-speed cycle on a box below parallel.

Week 1	330 lbs bar weight	440 lbs band tension	1 sets, 2 reps
Week 1	370 lbs bar weight	440 lbs band tension	1 sets, 2 reps
Week 1	420 lbs bar weight	440 lbs band tension	1 sets, 2 reps
Week 1	435 lbs bar weight	440 lbs band tension	1 sets, 1 reps
Week 2	330 lbs bar weight	440 lbs band tension	1 sets, 2 reps
Week 2	370 lbs bar weight	440 lbs band tension	1 sets, 2 reps
Week 2	420 lbs bar weight	440 lbs band tension	1 sets, 2 reps
Week 2	450 lbs bar weight	440 lbs band tension	1 sets, 1 reps

This is a continuation of three cycles. This first three-week wave is repeated in the second three-week wave followed by a two-week strength wave cycle. The strength-speed cycle should only last for two weeks because of its severity.

17. Arnold Coleman is an 876-lb squatter at a body weight of 181 lbs using a speed-strength workout with the lightened method.

Week 1	550 lbs bar weight	150 lbs lightened in hole	10 sets, 2 reps
Week 2	600 lbs bar weight	150 lbs lightened in hole	8 sets, 2 reps
Week 3	650 lbs bar weight	150 lbs lightened in hole	6 sets, 2 reps
Week 4	550 lbs bar weight	90 lbs lightened in hole	10 sets, 2 reps
Week 5	600 lbs bar weight	90 lbs lightened in hole	8 sets, 2 reps
Week 6	650 lbs bar weight	90 lbs lightened in hole	6 sets, 2 reps
Week 7	550 lbs bar weight	60 lbs lightened in hole	10 sets, 2 reps
Week 8	600 lbs bar weight	60 lbs lightened in hole	8 sets, 2 reps
Week 9	650 lbs bar weight	60 lbs lightened in hole	6 sets, 2 reps

The lightened method was used for juniors in the Soviet Union for weightlifting and gymnastics, but we've found it very successful for our most advanced lifters.

You must change the bar speed in different positions, which effects the relationship between force and posture, because muscular strength varies over the full range of joint motion. For more information, see Science and Practice of Strength Training by V. M. Zatsiorsky (1995).

To develop speed-strength, strength-speed, or slow strength, a plan of at least three weeks must be implemented and rotated constantly. In addition, explosive strength with very light weights and a maximum speed for a fast rate of force development should be used. In the circa-max phase, near-maximal weights are repeated for one and two reps and are limited to seven lifts. The different bars are in line with the conjugate system of equipment rotation and volume intensity zones. In addition, the bar speed should be changed on the eccentric phase as well as the concentric phase.

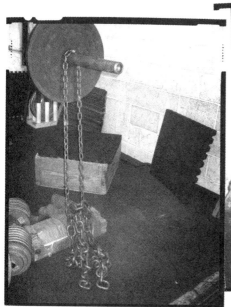

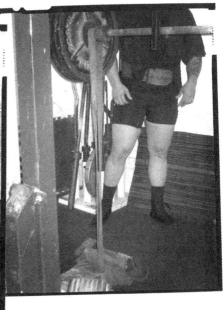

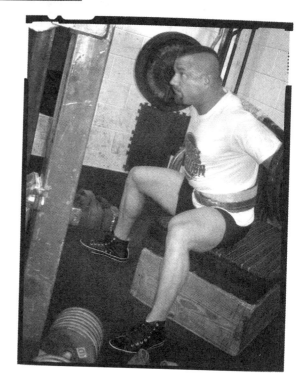

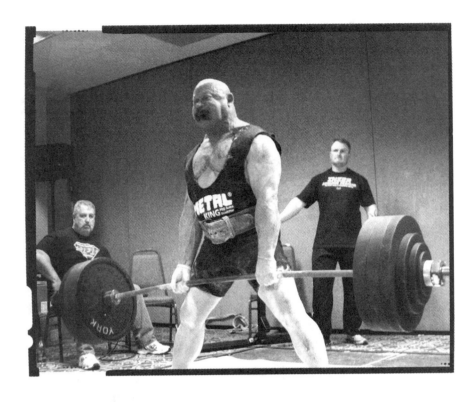

DEADLIFT TECHNIQUE

The great Mike Bridges said, "The deadlift is a squat with the bar in your hands." He's right.

Sumo Style

Just like in the power squat, push the feet apart and try to spread the floor. The knees should be over the bar to start the lift. Then, push your feet out to the sides to activate the hip muscles. The arms should hang straight down. Pull back while lifting the bar upward and push the knees out to help bring the hips toward the bar at lockout.

A reverse grip works for most individuals, but an overhand hook grip is best. It is difficult to manage though. The knee flexors help in the start of the deadlift, and the hips and glutes play a great role in locking out the lift. The squat and deadlift use the same muscles, but the main advantage in the deadlift is arm length.

Conventional Style

Foot spacing can range from heels touching to shoulder width apart. The heels together style places a large load on the hamstrings. The shoulder width style utilizes longer leg drive and more leg drive. The air should be in the stomach, not in the lungs. This will keep the torso as short as possible for better leverage. The knees should be over the bar at the start to ensure a powerful knee drive. A long-legged, short-back lifter will have the bar closest to his or her ankles. A short-legged, long-back lifter will sometimes place the bar at the center of the joint of the big toe.

The overhand hook grip is the best, but it's uncomfortable. A reverse palm grip is most common. The arms and upper back should be as relaxed as possible to shorten the pull. Always pull the bar toward the body. All pendulums act on their center of mass, and your arms can swing like a pendulum. Upon lifting the bar off of the floor, pull back as well as up. If you wait too long to pull back, it can lead to failure at lockout. Toes out equals a strong start. Toes straight equals a strong lockout.

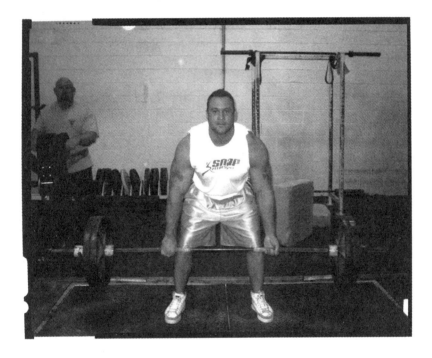

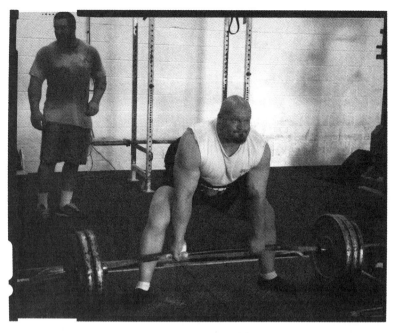

I hope a few tips can help correct your problems.

If you're weak off the floor, work on your abdominals and do knee extensions. Work on your start technique.

If you're weak at the knees, build your lower back. This is where the bar can be the furthest away from the hip joints.

If you're weak at lockout, do a lot of glute and hip work. All you have to do for locking out a deadlift is lean back and extend the hips. This is done with strong hips and glutes.

Work on hip flexibility by doing reverse hypers, pulling a sled, and pulling extra-wide sumo base deadlifts.

Notes for Squatting

Perform box squats as wide as possible. For meets, bring your stance in to build your squat mechanism and technique and use a box much lower than normal. You must fully sit back and then down to reach the box. After releasing the hip muscles, rock forward and use your back muscles first to raise yourself up. Use a wide stance to make balancing yourself difficult, which will teach you to place your weight on the center arch of the foot.

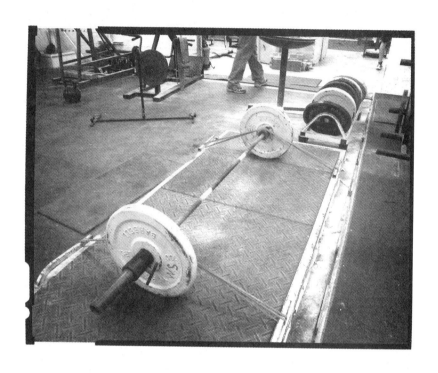

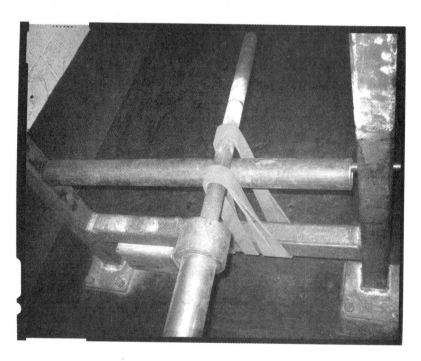

DEADLIFT PERIODIZATION

The deadlift and squat on max effort (ME) days are trained using the same exercises performed on Monday 72 hours after speed–strength, or dynamic day. An extreme workout can be performed every 72 hours, and a small workout or general physical preparedness (GPP) can be performed every 12–24 hours.

R otate a max squat exercise on ME day to a deadlift of some kind on the following Monday. Subsequently, perform a good morning of some kind on the following Monday on max effort day.

The max effort method is superior to all other training methods, but it's hard to maintain. Training the same exercise at 90 percent will eventually decrease progress or even cause regression. However, by rotating the bar exercise each week, this phenomenon can be eliminated. The body will only respond to the demands placed upon it. This means that whoever trains the heaviest most often will be the strongest.

As for the organization and periodization, it is truly a weekly plan. We plan during the week or sometimes at breakfast. At times, we even plan after arriving at the gym. In my opinion, long-term periodization is a mistake. I don't have a crystal ball to tell where someone's progress will be in 10, 16, or 52 weeks, so we do what needs to be done at the precise time we need it.

On a speed-strength day for squatting, we do speed pulls for 6–10 singles with 220 lbs of band tension at the top. Sometimes we do 5–10 sets of three reps in the power rack with 250–350 lbs of band tension. We always use conventional style deadlifts.

Currently, we're doing a much larger load of deadlifting to ensure better form and stronger grip. Our ability to pull a heavy deadlift at our meets has made it possible to win when we would have otherwise lost before from the lack of conditioning. You see, it is a plan without planning.

Strength is measured in time, not the weight lifted. We can only produce maximum muscle tension for a certain time limit. If the lift isn't completed in that time, you will fail. This style of ME periodization is a mixture of the Soviet system for Olympic lifting and the Bulgarian weightlifting system combined with my 43 years of powerlifting experience and shared knowledge with many of the greatest powerlifting minds of today.

My friend Sakari says it doesn't do any good to be good on the wrong lifts. Enough said.

Chapter 17

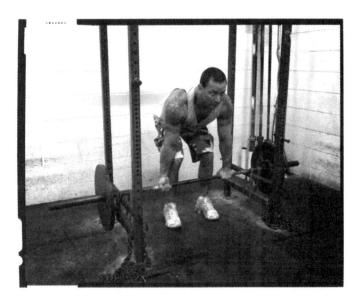

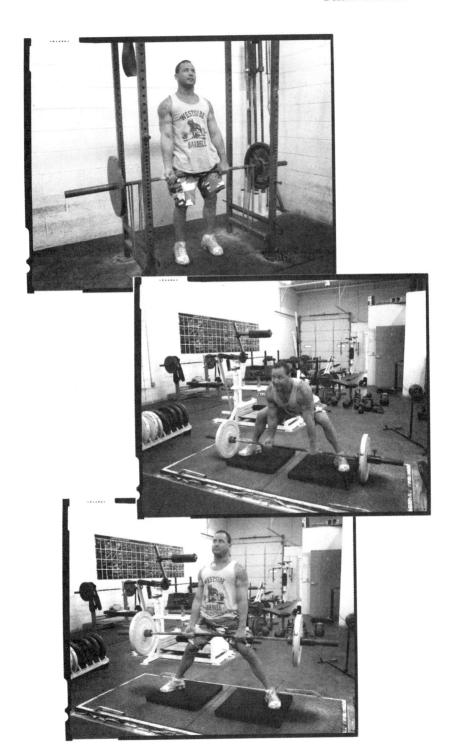

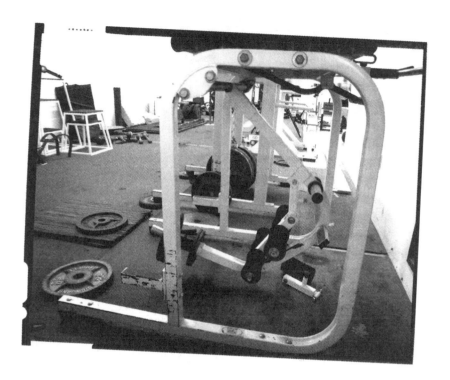

ELIMINATING WEAKNESSES

Muscular and Technical Weaknesses

As a lifter, you must learn good technical skills in the squat and deadlift at the very beginning. It doesn't matter if you squat using a close or wide stance or pull using the sumo or conventional style.

You must do certain mechanical movements with the proper joint movement at the right time. This can be accomplished by building the critical muscle groups, including the hips, upper and lower back, legs (front and back), and abs. For example, the abdominal muscles must be strong because you flex them first.

Many times when technique fails, your muscles fail first. These two weaknesses are often separated, but many times they go together. Everyone can do picture perfect squats and deadlifts with an empty bar.

Here are some common muscular and technical weaknesses in the squat:

- If your knees go forward, your glutes and hamstrings are weak and you're relying on your quads too much.

- If your knees come in, your hips are weak.

- If you bend over in the squat, your stomach and lower back are weak.

- If the weights feel heavy on your back, your traps and upper back are weak.

For squatting, if you don't sit back first, your glutes need more work.

- If you don't push your knees out while taking the bar out of the rack, your hips need more work.

- If you tilt forward while overcoming the weight, you are pushing with the feet first when you must push against the bar first.

- If you round over in the bottom of a squat, your upper back and abs are possibly weak or you are pushing with the feet first before pushing against the bar.

- While squatting, if you can't break parallel, you're not pushing your feet apart or your hips are weak.

Here are some common muscular and technical weaknesses in the deadlift:

- If your knees come in while sumo deadlifting, either you aren't pushing your feet apart while starting the bar off of the floor or your hips are weak and you can't push your feet apart because of weak hip muscles.

- If you can't lock out a deadlift, most think of an upper back issue and sometimes they're right. But it can also be weak hips that aren't allowing you to push to the proper hip extension, or you possibly lack hip flexibility.

- If you deadlift conventionally and you stiff leg your deadlifts unintentionally, you lack strong knee extension. This can lead to a back injury because you're overloading one area. Do box deadlifts on a two- to four-inch box. They can teach you to use your legs first, which is proper form. This will also build drive because you'll have to extend your legs the extra 2–4 inches.

What's the answer to muscular and technical weaknesses? You must make the posterior chain stronger. Glute ham raises, reverse hypers, and weighted sled pulls will build the calves, hamstrings, glutes, and hips.

Hanging leg raises and sit-ups, especially the straight leg type, will build the abdominals, and lat work like shrugs will build the upper back. Strong muscles will perfect your technique. This is just a small part of the conjugant system.

Here are some exercises that will correct the technical weaknesses for each muscle group.

Hips

- Sled pulls, front and sideways

- Wide stance low box squats

- Reverse hypers

- Ultra-wide sumo deadlifts

- Knee push aparts with jump stretch bands

- Walking with ankle weights of 20 lbs or more per leg

- Glute ham raises

- Good mornings, especially with bands

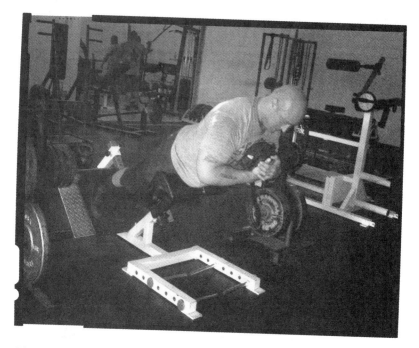

Hamstrings

• Glute ham raises

• Reverse hypers

• Sled pulls with strap held between legs, walking forward

• Band leg curls

• Good mornings of all types

• Wide stance squatting on a variety of box heights

• Ankle weight leg curls

Abdominals

- Stand up abdominals

- Straight leg sit-ups

- Leg raises

- Foam roller sit-ups

- Side bends

- One arm deadlifts sumo style

- Stand up static abdominal work

- Kettlebell work

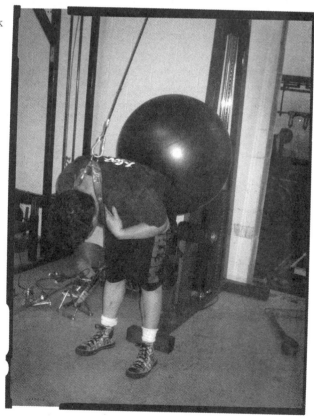

Spinal erectors

- Back extensions

- 45-degree back raises

- Reverse hypers

- Good mornings of all types

- All squatting

- All deadlifts of any style

- Kettlebell swings and cleans

- High-rep, low-intensity sled pulls

- Light leg curls for soft tissue training

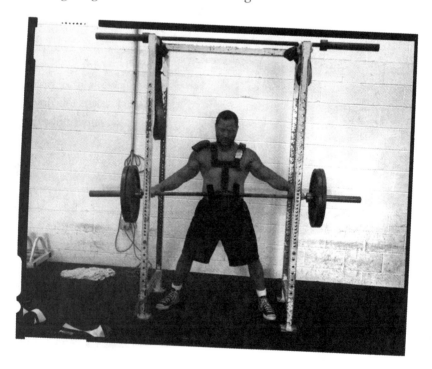

Mental Weaknesses

A high volume of training loads is a must to cause muscular and technical skill changes in a lifter, but sometimes it can be very stressful. Sometimes problems can occur, which show up as a lack of coordination. This is the ability to perform complex movements precisely and quickly (Science of Sports Training, Kurz).

But what do you do if you're mentally weak? Studies show that lifters should practice mental skills 3–5 times a week (Novicki, 1997).

Practice mental imaginary before bed and after waking up. If you fall asleep quickly, you're fatigued. If you're distracted and have trouble falling asleep, your schedule is too full. For more information, see Science of Sports Training by Thomas Kurz. If you aren't motivated, you could be in an overtrained state.

To build mental toughness for competitions, you must compete often and test yourself in training or tryouts. Challenge yourself with exercises you aren't good at or compete against someone who constantly beats you by a small margin.

By raising your pain tolerance, you will always hurt a little, but you must get used to it to reach the top. Learn to control your emotional state. Combat pain and overcome fear by relaxation, hypnotism, mental imaginary, and confidence in your skills.

Sticking Point Elimination

Your sticking point, or mini-max, is precisely where you can execute minimal force against max resistance loading to joint angles. This represents the peak contraction principle and is the weakest point of the human strength curve (Science and Practice of Strength Training, V.M. Zatriorsky).

There are three ways to combat sticking points:

1. The already mentioned peak contraction principle

2. Accentuation, where one works precisely within the range of main sport movement

3. Accommodation (Bands and chains will add extra resistance when joint angles have improved the relationship between force and posture.)

We use all three, but accommodation by resistance is used the most.

There's also bar speed. For example, if your sticking point in the deadlift is four inches off of the floor with 800 lbs, why don't you get stuck at four inches off the floor with 700 lbs? You don't get stuck because the barbell is moving fast enough through the sticking point.

So the answer to this mini-max is bar speed. It is increased with the dynamic method. Force equals mass times acceleration. Think about the three ways to combat sticking points and decide for yourself.

Chapter 18

PREPARING FOR A CONTEST

Contest preparation at Westside lasts 5–6 weeks. The circa-max wave lasts three weeks, the upward wave lasts two weeks, and one week is for deloading. The final week is the most important—the contest.

S quat training is on Fridays. When preparing for a contest, the first week consists of 6–8 lifts between 90–97 percent of a one rep max. For example, an 800-lb squatter would do 370 lbs for two reps, 420 lbs for two reps, 460 lbs for two reps, and 480 lbs for one rep. The bar also has strong Jump Stretch bands that supply 340–375 lbs of tension at lockout.

During the second week, the lifter will do 370 lbs for two reps, 420 lbs for two reps, 470 lbs for one rep, and sometimes over 500 lbs for a new one rep max.

Week three is a download of intensity and volume. After a warmup, the lifter will do three singles with 370–420 lbs and one with 470 lbs. That concludes the circa-max phase.

Mondays are max effort days for the squat and deadlift, but during the squat circa-max phase, the max effort day is converted to repetition work, concentrating on the reverse hypers, glute ham raises, back raises, lots of upper back work, and most importantly, sled pulling for restoration.

During this monthly cycle, the weights above 90 percent are transferred to Friday's squat workout. The deadlifts are speed pulls and are done on the Friday immediately after circa-max squats.

Using the box squat, here are some examples of what to expect at a contest:

- 800-lb squat —   500 lbs plus 340 lbs of bands at top

- 850-lb squat —   556 lbs plus 340 lbs of bands at top

- 900-lb squat —   600 lbs plus 340 lbs of bands at top

- 950-lb squat —   660 lbs plus 340 lbs of bands at top

- 1000-lb squat —   620 lbs plus 440 lbs of bands at top

- 1050-lb squat —   660 lbs plus 440 lbs of bands at top

These examples have been proven over and over at Westside by lifters who are five feet, six inches in height and taller.

Dynamic Contest Preparation

Using three sets of chains for a total of 120 lbs added to the bar, three men performed their first 800-lb squats officially.

Week 1: 50% of 400 lbs x 2 reps x 12 sets = 9600 lbs

Week 2: 55% of 440 lbs x 2 reps x 12 sets= 10,560 lbs

Week 3: 60% of 480 lbs x 2 reps x 12 sets= 9600 lbs

Week 4: 50% of 400 lbs x 1 rep x 5 sets = 2000 lbs

Week four is a deload or short delayed transformation phase. This allows the lifters to recover from the previous training.

The final week is of course the meet. We suggest you start around 90 percent of your best squat. This system works well for those who like high volume with lots of bar speed. A single with 700 lbs will most often render an 800-lb contest squat after the straps are pulled up and the knee wraps are added.

After adding four sets of $^5/_8$-inch chains totaling 160 lbs to the bar, three men performed their first 900-lb squats officially.

Week 1: 50% of 450 lbs x 2 reps x 12 sets = 10,800 lbs

Week 2: 55% of 495 lbs x 2 reps x 12 sets = 11,880 lbs

Week 3: 60% of 540 lbs x 2 reps x 10 sets = 10,800

Week 4: 65% of 450 lbs x 1 rep x 5 sets = 2250 lbs

For the last week before contest day, use the same procedures as for an 800-lb open at close to 90 percent.

Proper form must be used on the box as well as on contest day. A regular squat on meet day should be easy after box squatting. By adding wraps, putting your straps up, and not pausing in the bottom, you should get a huge carryover from the box to contest squatting.

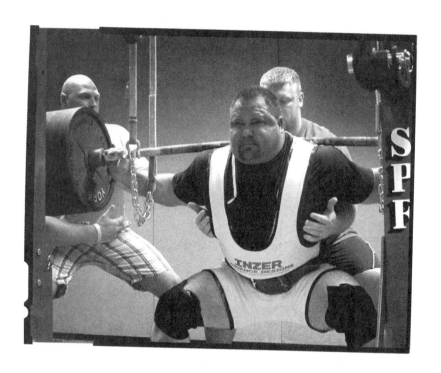

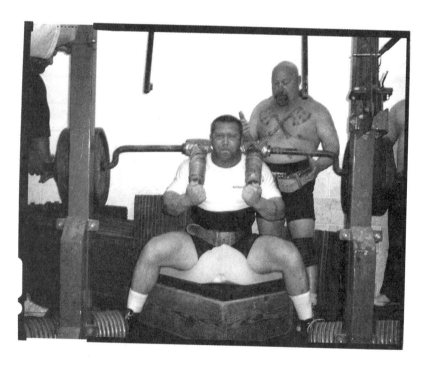

GEAR TRAINING FOR THE SQUAT AND DEADLIFT

How does Westside use supportive gear in training and for competition?

For speed squatting on Fridays, we warm up to about 40 percent of a one rep max without gear. As the weight goes up, briefs must be worn.

Personally, I use one of four pairs of briefs. If the working sets are light, I use the least supportive pair. As the working set becomes harder, I go for the next pair of briefs for more support. This is for speed-strength sets. As we enter into strength-speed or circa-max weight, I bring out the stronger pairs. As the weights move up to maxes, I add one of three suits over the briefs. My poly suit is less resistive. When the weights grow for the next workout, I wear a light canvas over my strongest briefs. When it is time to take an all-time record, I wear the strongest briefs and my strongest suit—an Inzer Leviathan canvas.

Too much gear will hinder your form. You won't be able to sit back, push your knees apart, or keep your knees from pushing forward, all of which is very dangerous. However, if you don't have enough gear, you may not be able to handle the desired weight.

You must learn what combination is best for what amount of resistance you're using. And you must wear gear to become a top ten lifter. By wearing a power belt, you might be able to squat or deadlift an additional 50–100 lbs. A belt only covers four inches of your body, but that four-inch belt is making the other lifters' bodies do that extra 50–100 lbs. Just think what a pair of briefs could do! If you think the brief is allowing you to lift let's say 150 lbs, why don't your lower leg muscles or back muscles succumb to the extra stress? It is because of intermuscular coordination and the demand placed on the central nervous system.

Gear for the Meet

We almost never use top gear in training with knee wraps and the suit straps up. Why? If your form is good, gear will make it better. If your form is bad, gear will make it worse. So learn to box squat correctly and your regular squat form will be perfect. A box squat is much harder than a contest style squat.

Over the years, we have had fifteen 1000-lb squatters and four squatters who did over 1100 lbs. I don't know a gym that can duplicate this.

Wearing straps up and knee wraps will enable you to lift a lot in the squat, but it seems to hinder deadlift progress somewhat. We very seldom put the straps up in the lightened method. Much of our deadlift max effort training is performed in regular gym shorts plus a belt. We only use our briefs on sumo pulls, and none of our small exercises, including glute ham raises, reverse hypers, sled pulls, and wheelbarrows, are done with gear.

This, I believe, is why we have 15 members with an 800-lb deadlift or higher plus six women with a deadlift over 500 lbs.

While in the gym, briefs or a suit may be used but never with the straps up. The straps will give you some amount of carryover for the meet.

My friend Eskil Thomasson was out of meets for four years due to some lagging knee injuries. He never wore his straps up or knee wraps in that four years, but upon his return to the platform, he hit an all-time squat record plus a deadlift record. Enough said?

Remember, wear strong gear in training when the intensity calls for it. It is important on the eccentric phase to duplicate the slower eccentric phase that is caused by tight wraps and the strongest suit possible at the meet.

A final note: most have to use a closer stance in meets compared to the box squat stance. It is easier to use optimal eccentrics on a box due to less gear. This is why you must use a closer stance for a meet.

Training and Meet Coaching Tips

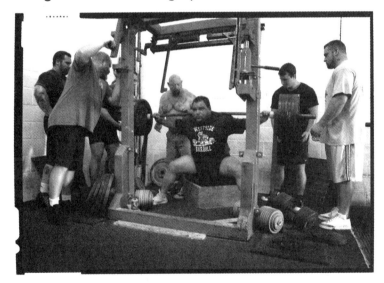

Coaching is irritating with very light weights, but when you reach roughly 50 percent of a one rep max, you should start coaching. Just don't overcoach. In the gym, you should be instructed to arch the bar out of the back. Don't push up with the legs but rather push out to the sides to ensure that your hips are activated fully. Pick up the chest, pull the elbows forward, and arch the upper back. This is most important because that is where the bar sits, and the bar is what you are trying to move. On the eccentric phase, the coach should instruct the lifter to push the glutes out to the rear as the knees and hips are forced out to the sides. By doing this, it shortens the distance the bar moves eccentrically and concentrically. It makes breaking parallel easier. The feet should also be pushed outward, not down. This will produce more force. As a coach, I recommend Chuck Taylor shoes. Mel Siff once said that the best shoe is no shoe.

Don't carry the bar too low because it will actually cause you to lean over and lose power, which makes it difficult to break parallel because of the excessive lean. You'll end up not going lower but forward, keeping the hips above parallel. A low bar on your back also makes it difficult to lock out the squat. There are rules about the bar position on the back that make it illegal to place the bar too low. But rule or no rule, it's a bad idea. It is very hard on the bicep tendons and shoulders as well. How you take the bar out of the rack is how you will squat. If you take it out correctly, you will squat correctly. If you take it out incorrectly, you will squat incorrectly. It's that simple.

A coach must be sure the lifter is doing speed sets with perfect form. If not, it will show up with the heavier weights. If your special exercises are going up but your squat isn't, your form has a flaw or possibly a weak muscle group has eluded you.

Deadlift Coaching

A conventional deadlifter must learn to stand a proper distance from the bar. If you're too far away, the bar will swing toward you, which will cause you to bend over too much. Large men and women often stand too close to the bar, which causes the bar to swing forward and past the knees. These are the two most common flaws at the start.

Most deadlifters use leg drive at the start and pull backward to some extent. All objects will swing toward the center mass point. If your feet point straight forward, you'll have a strong finish. If your toes are turned out, you'll develop a strong start.

As for grip, a double, overhand hook grip is best, but few can master it. The most common and effective grip is one palm forward and one palm backward. Nonetheless, a strong grip is a must for a great deadlift. Don't wear straps if possible. Experiment with the foot stance and grip width. When pulling off the floor and driving the legs at the same time, the tension should be felt in the hands. If you're only using leg drive, your deadlift will result in a miss at knee level. All the tension in the hands will cause you to round over due to lack of leg drive.

Sumo Deadlift Coaching Tips

The stance is optional, but the wider it is, the more hip action you'll need. The closer you are to the bar, the more leg drive you'll need. Always push the feet apart and never down. The main key is to push the feet apart and pull the bar toward the body. Mike Bridges said that a sumo deadlift is just a squat with a bar in the hands. It's that simple if you have good squat form. Don't overdo it with the gear. You must be able to get in the proper starting position. There are many suits to choose from so experiment. There isn't any one best suit for squatting or deadlifting—only the best suit for you personally.

Squat Deadlift Cycling

After speed squatting on Friday, where we do several sets with short rest periods, we immediately go to speed pulls for 5–10 singles. We almost always do these with bands over the bar or 5–10 sets of rack pulls with bands for pause triples. This can be very taxing, but you will adapt. This day has a large volume of moderate intensity zones and is a must to wave the volume downward greatly but raise the intensity to 100 percent or more on max effort day. The squatting and combined speed or rack pulls or Friday's high volume are waved upward in the squat but downward in the deadlift weight. Although bar speed may suffer somewhat on squatting, the deadlifts become faster. Wave training isn't found on max effort day but 72 hours later on Monday. The deadlift training is planned weekly, one week at a time. It could be a special squat, deadlift, good morning, or heavy sled pulls. Choose what is best for you.

Always train the small exercises in high volume after both days. As Sakari said, it does not help to be strong in the wrong exercise. Don't pull heavy three weeks before the meet. Most heavy work is done on Friday, which is squat day, during the circa-max phase. This means do the max effort exercises on Friday and leave Monday for the development of small muscle groups. Last but not least, don't forget restoration methods. The delayed transformation time lasts two weeks and then you have the meet, which is 21 days after the heaviest loads determined by the percentage of a one rep max.

WESTSIDE PLYOMETRICS – BOX JUMPING

Y. V. Verkoshansky, the father of plyometrics, discovered the phenomenon of the stretch reflex by watching triple jumpers perform. He was amazed by the powerful rebound on each preceding landing. Track and field and Olympic weightlifting have used the benefits of plyometrics for over four decades. Plyometrics can also elevate the standard for the power lifts.

Westside has done numerous experiments with jumping. Our goal was to jump on the highest box possible without resistance other than air and gravity. Working with NFL players, NFL combine candidates, Olympic sprinters, and of course, world class powerlifters, we have developed a system to improve the maximum rate of force development using revolving jump drills that have made it possible to attain a 60-inch box jump.

Box Squat Box Jump

Sitting on a box about three inches above parallel, lifting the feet off the ground, and slamming them down again while jumping has produced the best technique for increasing a long jump or box jump for height.

We know that as the lifter lowers himself onto the box, he represents potential energy. After contact with the box, he creates kinetic energy. The collision with the glutes and upper thighs isn't considered perfectly elastic but rather inelastic. Add this to the feet being slammed on the floor and a large amount of kinetic energy is produced. This leads to the most productive method for increasing jumping ability.

Pete Campion played as a lineman for five years for the NFL Raiders. A weekend visit to Westside earned him the longest long jump of his career. Pete had long jumped in high school and in the NFL, but in a span of 48 hours at Westside, he jumped further than ever before. How? By sitting on a 17-inch bench, rocking back and forth, picking up his feet, and then slamming them down before jumping forward.

Another example is a 292-lb tight end from the Mac conference who ran a 5.1-second 40-yard dash. I reduced his time to 4.9 seconds. After two months, he ran a 4.77-second 40 at his college professional tryout. The special jumping played a large role in his program. His school was an Olympic lifting school, and he had spent four years there wasting his time. Olympic lifting has very little to do with jumping. By the way, his long jump went from eight feet, nine inches to nine feet, eight inches. Everyone knows that we power lift. We don't run ball players but rather have them jump, power lift, and power walk with weight sleds. I won't name his school or the strength coaches' names, but he still does the same old program.

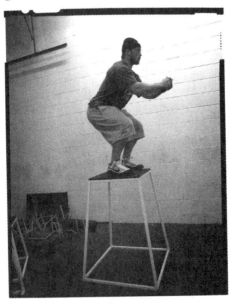

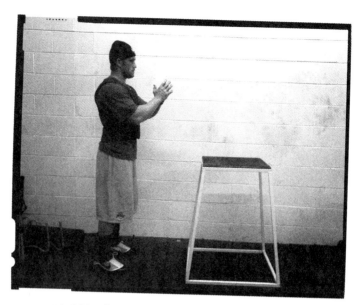

Jumping with Ankle Weights

Jumps with ankle weights ranging from 5–40 lbs per leg are done on a variety of boxes. Ankle weight jumps are done in sets of five jumps, and the emphasis is on strength. Thirty jumps are optimal with light weight. When using heavy ankle weights of 25–40 lbs, the jumps go down to 15 jumps. Single or double leg jumps should be altered.

Dumbbell Box Jumps

John Stafford has jumped onto a 36-inch box with a pair of 70-lb dumbbells at a body weight of 290 lbs. A 290-lb tight end made a 36-inch box jump with a pair of 60-lb dumbbells. Again, we aim for 15–30 box jumps per workout. Use a combination of ankle weights and dumbbells. Keep track of records of all types.

This type of dynamic loading can be very taxing. Limit the weight jumps to no less than 72 hours between workouts. If you do depth jumps, start from 12–20 inches. Depending on whether or not you're an advanced 800-lb or more squatter, raise the box to 30–40 inches and land on approximately a two-inch rubber mat. Drop straight down with your arms behind your body. After landing on the balls of your feet, lower onto the heels with your legs slightly bent. Swing your arms forward and jump upward explosively, landing in the same spot you jumped from. The amortization phase will vary depending on how far you bend at the knees.

Weight vests can be used for jumping up on boxes on a regular basis. But you should only jump off of a box from a soft surface. Of course, jumping without arm swings can be done or jumping upward without an eccentric phase. Jump squats or step-ups are also a valuable tool.

I prefer to do simple exercises for jumping. If jumping is that important—and it is—there should be special exercises to increase jumping. I am a fan and student of Starzynski and Sozanski. Check out the book Explosive Power and Jumping Ability for all Sports.

Why do strength and jumping go hand in hand? They go hand in hand because the maximal velocity that can be displayed in a given movement depends heavily on the level of strength first and then coordination, flexibility, and technical skills. Strength first? Yes. This can be explained by junior weightlifters outjumping junior jumpers in the first three years. I am not a big fan of Olympic lifts for sports. The push jerk or press is the only element that contributes to jumping by the creation of an amortizing phase. The support reaction in the phase is 233–245 percent of the bar weight, but I am a total believer in doing Olympic lifts from a seated knee position.

While in high school, John Harper of Cincinnati could jump onto his feet from a sitting position on the ground with 170 lbs on his back. As a junior in college, he could jump about 195 feet. At this point, he could jump onto his feet with 265 lbs at a body weight of 265 lbs.

Our Sequence

1. Sit on the floor with your legs straight in front of you. Place a barbell on your upper thigh. Clean and press a bar over your head for several sets of 5–10 reps. Beginners should use several sets of 3–8 reps. Take rest breaks to ensure optimal recovery.

2. Sit up on the knees. Sit back onto your glutes and jump onto your feet. After mastering this, place a barbell on your back and jump onto your feet. Later, jump up into a jump squat.

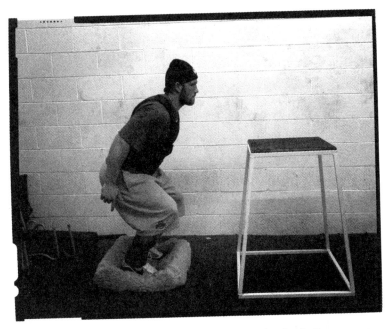

3. Sit on the knees, and sit back on the glutes with a barbell across the upper thighs. Jump up into a power clean.

4. Sit on your knees and then lower onto your glutes with a barbell across the upper thighs. Do a power snatch.

5. Sit on the knees, lower onto your glutes with a barbell across your thighs, and do a split snatch. Alternate for each leg.

It is best to do repetitions with the above exercises. Multiple jumps can be a common means of increasing jumping ability in all sports. These multi-jumps will increase jumping endurance, jumping ability, and sport-specific strength (Mroczynski and Starzynski, 1994).

I suggest jump roping first for timing, rhythm, and endurance. Master the kneeling jumps without weight first. These jumps are primarily for squatting and pulling power as well as increasing vertical jumping and box jumping ability. For long jumping, jump from the kneeling position without weight at first onto a low box. Our top jumpers can land on a 14-inch box from the knees. These jumps build a maximal rate of force development.

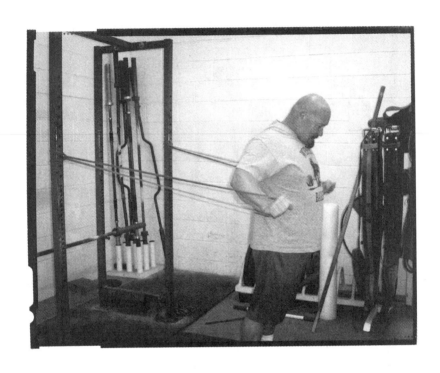

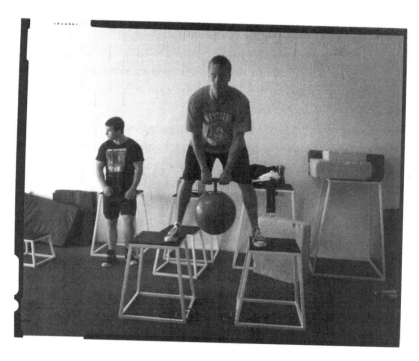

SPECIAL EXERCISES – ASSISTANCE WORK

Exercises can fall into three categories: general, directed, and sports-specific.

G eneral exercises include the reverse hypers, glute ham raises, box jumps, inverse curls, lat work, abdominal work, triceps extensions, and hip extensor/flexor work.

Directed exercises include good mornings, belt squats, floor presses, rack or board presses, dumbbell presses, and deadlifts on a box or from a rack.

Sports-specific exercises include legal depth box squats, close grip bench presses, and wide bench presses as well as deadlifting with the opposite style that you normally use (sumo versus conventional).

At Westside, all three categories are used each week. They aren't done simultaneously. Why? If a specific type of strength isn't trained during a three-week period, a loss in strength of 10 percent or greater occurs. This is true for agility, coordination, and even flexibility.

Small Exercises for the Squat and Deadlift

Upper back and lats:

- Reverse bench pull downs

- Low pull downs

- Dumbbell rows

- Barbell rows

- Chest-supported rows

- T-bar rows

- Chin-ups

- Sled lat pulls

Lower back:

- Reverse hypers

- 45-degree hypers

- Back raises

- Inverse curls

- Kettlebell deadlifts

- Back Attack

- Bent over sled pulls

Abdominal exercises:

- Crunches

- Sit-ups of all kinds

- Stand up abs

- Leg raises sitting down

- Hanging leg raises

- Walking with leg weights

- Stand up abs

- Stability ball sit-ups

Hamstring exercises:

- Glute ham raises

- Leg curls on the machine

- Leg curls with ankle weights

- Stiff leg deadlifts

- Reverse hypers

Trap exercises:

- Dumbbell shrugs

- Barbell shrugs

- High pulls

- Snatch grips

- Clean grips

- Shrugs behind back

GPP, SPP, AND HYPERTROPHY

General physical preparedness (GPP) must be a priority in your training in order to reach the top. A lifter must recover from workout to workout. As the training becomes harder and more intense, better recovery methods must be employed. These can include flexibility, mobility, speed, and endurance work. Sometimes perfecting form or receiving massages, water therapy, or electrostimulation can aid in recovery as well. Lifters should use all rehabilitation procedures available. Lifters' blood pressure and pulse should be tracked at all times to determine their trainability. If you don't have a plan, you plan to fail.

It is common to see lifters at Westside pulling a light sled with one or two 45-lb plates for up to three-quarters of a mile or walking while wearing weight vests with up to 100 lbs for a mile. Lifters also walk with 10–40-lb ankle weights for half a mile or walk with a Zercher harness and up to 135 lbs for a quarter mile at a time for a total of a half mile. Use combinations of any of these. Westside also uses a nonmotorized treadmill known as the Tred Sled. With this device, we attach bands around the waist or ankles. We also use 25–50-lb vests and ankle weights of varying weights. Any combination of resistance can be used.

GPP can be included for bounding and jumping exercises. Long jumps, triple long jumps, and box jumps should be performed on a regular basis. Try adding ankle weights, weight vests, dumbbells, or a combination of all three. You can also jump while standing on foam. Try sitting on a lower box and jumping onto another predetermined box. This works well for standing long jumps as well. Remember, jumping rope is the most basic plyometric drill.

Many of our powerlifters have football backgrounds at the high school or college level. Jim Wendler comes to mind. He played at Arizona as a fullback and was one of the most explosive lifters I have ever seen. He went on to squat 1000 lbs, and it was explosive. I surmise it was part genetics and a larger part GPP from his sport background.

GPP should occur in the early stages of training prior to specialization training for a particular sport. It is intended to develop general jumping, coordination, endurance, flexibility, and strength training. If a youth is pushed into sports, barriers can occur. The most common is the so-called speed barrier. This means that an athlete learns to move at a certain speed but no faster. The central nervous system will automatically move at a certain speed and develop frequency standards. Doing more of the same work won't help. Instead, it exacerbates the problem. The fix is to use new stimulants to bring about new results and make the athlete forget his physical and mental barriers.

At Westside, we use sled pulling for general conditioning as well as for strength training and restoration work.

It is commonly used for a warmup and to raise a lifter's aerobic capabilities and work the cardiovascular system. For maximal strength work, we pull a sled hooked to a power belt by a strap and walk forward and backward for distances of 100 feet to one mile. Pulls for longer distances can be used for restoration and general endurance. By pulling with the straps backward between the legs, you can work the hamstrings as well as get great hip and knee extension. You can also work the muscles of the upper body by using the upper body more when pulling the sled.

For greater intensity, pull the sled while wearing a weight vest up to 150 lbs. Walk forward, backward, and even sideways for a quarter mile to one and a half miles, depending on your abilities. This is also a great way to warm up for squatting, deadlifting, or even benching. Just cut the distance back to a quarter of a mile or a half mile.

Wearing ankle weights is a great form of conditioning. Place an ankle weight of about 5 lbs on each ankle and wear them around the gym or for a brisk walk. Work up to a top weight of 20 lbs for each leg. Yes, this means 40 lbs for both legs. Besides building the legs and abdominals, ankle weights also traction out the knees, hips, and lower back. Hand weights, kettlebells, and Indian clubs can accompany the ankle weights. If you want a very difficult workout, pull a sled while wearing a weight vest and ankle weights and carrying kettlebells.

Other great forms of general conditioning or GPP include kettlebells and wheelbarrow walking. The latter is great for the hips and legs, and the distance is calculated by the weight of the load. At Westside, we perform high-rep leg curls with ankle weights on a regular basis. The hamstrings can be a troublesome area, and the high-rep conditioning has proven to be a very effective method for avoiding hamstring pulls. We also take short walks, and there's even a mountain bike to ride at Westside.

The best GPP training I've found is sled work for both the upper and lower body. But how much GPP is too much and how do you know if you're getting too little? How do you taper the volume, and how high should the intensity be?

There are four training periods to cycle in and out of:

Accumulation: Lifters must include as much work in this cycle as possible. A high training volume is effective at this stage, and a manageable intensity zone must be planned by the lifter or coach, meaning loads that can be repeated fairly easily can be performed for some predetermined time. All muscle groups must be trained. Powerlifters must work on increasing the bar speed, eliminating technical weaknesses, and of course, raising GPP.

Intensification: At this stage, you must eliminate some exercises and concentrate on the main task. For example, cut back on belt squatting and raise the amount of box squatting per week and per month, or cut back on slow deadlifts such as rack pulls and concentrate more on speed pulls. Eliminate some types of sled pulls by decreasing the number of trips or the weight. Or do only the lat exercise that works best for you in volume and number of reps and concentrate more on full-range pulling.

Transformation: This is the stage when the lifter evaluates the two previous periodizations. The lifter selects the power lifts, the box squat, and the deadlift along with three or four special exercises that work best for him. Doing the wrong exercises won't work. Be sure that your selections will make you stronger for contest day. This will prevent overtraining. While performing the heaviest training, commonly known as the circa-max phase, proper restoration methods will play an important role during the last training phase. In addition, check your nutrition plan. It is important to pay attention to nutrition throughout the year, but it's very important during the transformation phase.

Delayed transformation: This is a tapering down phase that should last 14–21 days from a contest of high importance. The total volume and intensity zone are lowered considerably from the previous training periods. A lifter must be fully recovered on competition day. This is a guideline that Westside follows, and so far it has produced eleven 2500-lb totals and five 2600-lb totals. By using the conjugate system, everything will fall together. You will be more muscular, faster, and better conditioned, and most importantly, you will be stronger. More information can be found in The Science of Sports Training by Thomas Kurz and Science and Practice of Strength Training by V. M. Zatsiorsky.

RESTORATION

A lifter needs adequate recovery to reach his potential. Seventy-two hours between extreme workouts is optimal. Smaller workouts can occur 12–24 hours apart. At Westside, we choose the exercises for each workout carefully. This keeps overtraining at bay. Westside has followed the reasoning of Olympic-caliber weightlifters. Their heavy squat workouts are 72 hours apart. This approach has Westside squatting on Friday with moderately high intensity and high volume.

Max effort day—Monday—is 72 hours later. The intensity is high and the volume is low. It looks like a contest with one lift at around 90 percent and one just under or just over an all-time best. Your level of preparedness will decide if you break your all-time record or not. Remember to switch a major barbell exercise each week, and always vary the volume and intensities in each workout.

Some common restoration methods include:

Ice bath (apply ice to an overstressed muscle group)

Hot tub (alternate with ice or cold baths)

Dry sauna

Wet heat

Laser biostimulation

Electrostimulation

Hand sport massage

Deep tissue rolfing

Static and dynamic stretching (to improve flexibility and aid in range of motion)

Chiropractic and traction devices as well as adequate sleep and proper nutrition can help in restoration. Sufficient protein, vitamins, and minerals are essential. You must take advantage of everything at your disposal. Even a small walk can help restore your body for the next workout or help you shed a few pounds. Remember, relaxation can play a large role in restoration as well.

It's important to get chiropractic adjustments, especially for the neck. Proper spinal alignment will eliminate some hamstring pulls and help relieve IT band tightness. Heavy squats and good mornings could cause trauma to the upper back, causing pain and weakness. Sometimes this pain travels down to the fingertips and can cause weakness and numbness in the grip.

Restoration can and should be low intensity. Walking is great restoration, but, as the saying goes, I like to kill two birds with one stone. During the morning workout, I pull a light sled with 45–90 lbs for 6–10 trips of 60 yards. This is great for both the lower body and upper body muscle groups. You will suffer from accommodation if you continue to do the same work at the same intensity and volume.

When you've done the light sled work for awhile, increase the distance to two miles or wear ankle weights or a weight vest. You can rotate this exercise with a special non-motorized treadmill and wear a weight vest or ankle weights for resistance. This workout will take no more than 20 minutes and will be much more intense than just walking outside. Many more steps are done per minute on the non-motorized treadmill. Another option is wheelbarrow walking. Try walking forward or backward like a rickshaw. This is great for overall conditioning as well.

Don't underestimate kettlebell work of all types. I've cleaned a 16-kg kettlebell for 15 minutes, continuously rotating from my left arm to the right. I consider this a type of restoration. You can also try alternating-arm snatches with light kettlebells. Just pick something you can do for at least five minutes. I've cleaned a 24-kg kettlebell for five minutes, but that is considered a strength endurance workout because it is much too taxing for restoration. Although they are intertwined, don't confuse the two.

Swimming is a great form of restoration because the water provides resistance. I can't swim, but I do 200–500 kick steps in a pool much like V. Alexeev, who did 1000 per day for hip and abdominal strength to prevent injury. You can also try doing 300 triceps push-downs during the week outside the gym by placing a light band over a door at home. Do 100 reps at a time for a total of 300 reps. Leg curls with bands or ankle weights should be done as well. Although I've mentioned this several times, Diane Guthrie does 250 leg curls a day with 10-lb ankle weights. She stopped doing them for a period of time and hurt her leg muscles. She started the leg curls again and eliminated her injury.

We believe in three-week waves for strength. Studies (L. P. Matveeve 1980) have shown that lifters have physical biocycles lasting 23 days, which falls in line perfectly with our three-week wave.

Never do a restoration GPP cycle that lasts longer than 23 days.

As far as recovery goes, don't leave any stone unturned. There are many more methods that I haven't discussed, but I hope I've made you think about how you can make progress when you aren't in the weight room. The higher the mental demands that you place on yourself, the shorter the restoration cycle. This information should help you reach your strength and fitness potential

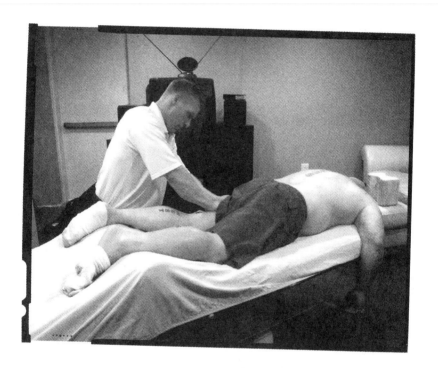

WESTSIDE STATS FOR THE SQUAT AND DEADLIFT

Top Ten Squats

Rank	Last name	First Name	Total (lbs)	Weight class	BW (lbs)	Coefficient
1	Vogelpohl	Chuck	1150	275	264	606.4
2	Bolognone	Tony	1150	308	300	583,9
3	Alhazov	Vlad	1155	shw	341	579,5
4	Panora	Greg	1060	242	242	568,6
5	Hoff	Dave	1075	275	275	568,2
6	Vogelpohl	Chuck	1025	220	220	567,8
7	Harrington	Phil	905	181	181	560,46
8	Roberts	AJ	1100	308	300	558,03
9	Harrington	Phil	945	198	197	554,6
10	Bolognone	Tony	1125	shw	332	553,38

SHW = Super heavyweight

Top Ten Deadlifts

Rank	Last name	First Name	Total (lbs)	Weight class	BW (lbs)	Coefficient
1	Vogelpohl	Chuck	816	220	220	452,06
2	Edwards	Luke	840	275	265	442,6
3	Vogelpohl	Chuck	835	275	265	439,62
4	Heath	Doug	540	132	132,25	438,9
5	Chorpenning	Jeff	750	198	198,5	438,8
6	Panora	Greg	815	242	242	437,2
7	Vogelpohl	Chuck	805	242	234	437,03
8	Hoff	Dave	825	242	262	435,8
9	Edwards	Luke	810	242	240	435,5
10	Heath	Doug	457	114	114,5	434,8

1100-lb Squat Club

Rank	Last name	First Name	Lift (lbs)	Weight class
1	Smith	Matt	1160	SHW
2	Alvazov	Vlad	1155	SHW
3	Vogelpohl	Chuck	1150	275
4	Bolognone	Tony	1150	308
5	Roberts	AJ	1100	308

SHW = Super heavyweight

1000-lb Squat Club

Rank	Last name	First Name	Lift (lbs)	Weight class
6	Hoff	Dave	1075	275
7	Brown	Mike	1074	308
8	Panora	Greg	1060	242

Rank	Last name	First Name	Lift (lbs)	Weight class
9	Wenning	Matt	1055	275
10	Anderson	Jake	1050	308
11	Ruggiera	Mike	1050	348
12	Cole	Zach	1040	308
13	Edwards	Luke	1025	242
14	Dimel	Matt	1010	SHW
15	Lily	Brandon	1005	308
16	Harold	Tim	1005	SHW
17	Wendler	Jim	1000	275

SHW = Super heavyweight

900-lb Squat Club

Rank	Last name	First Name	Lift (lbs)	Weight class
1	Harrington	Phil	960	220
2	Church	Shane	960	242
3	Meyers	Jeriamiah	950	275
4	Waddle	Tom	950	308
5	Stafford	John	946	275
6	Tate	Dave	935	308
7	Bayles	Joe	925	242
8	Burrows	Mark	925	275
9	Simmons	Louie	920	242
10	Henry	Andre	920	SHW
11	Fusner	Rob	905	308
12	Holdsworth	JL	903	275
13	Hudak	Zack	903	275
14	Nutter	Shawn	900	242

Rank	Last name	First Name	Lift (lbs)	Weight class
15	Douglas	Richard	900	275
16	Madjar	Matt	900	275
17	Ramsey	Will	900	308
18	Lenigar	Matt	900	308
19	Guttridge	Josh	900	SHW

SHW = Super heavyweight

800-lb Squat Club

Rank	Last name	First Name	Lift (lbs)	Weight class
1	Mendoza	Phil	881	SHW
2	Ritchey	Jimmy	875	275
3	Amato	Joe	865	275
4	Jester	Joe	860	220
5	Shackelford	John	850	242
6	Smith 2	Matt	850	242
7	Brock	Todd	850	275
8	Willoughby	Jerry	850	SHW
9	Thomasson	Eskil	840	242
10	Douglas	Rich	840	275
11	Youngs	Bob	840	308
12	Beach	Tony	830	308
12	McCoy	Joe	825	220
13	Blanton	mike	825	275
14	Patterson	Kenny	821	220
15	Brown	John	820	220
16	Reitter	Gabe	820	242
17	Ramos	Tony	815	181
18	Hayes	Bill	815	SHW

Rank	Last name	First Name	Lift (lbs)	Weight class
19	Hawkins	Matt	810	220
20	Obradovic	Jerry	810	275
21	Forby	Tim	810	308
22	Moore	Bill	805	SHW
23	Chorpenning	Jeff	804	198
24	Coleman	Arnold	804	198
25	Trotter	Rick	800	242
26	Henderson	Shawn	800	275
27	Johnson	Nate	800	275
28	Snyder	John	800	275
29	Damron	Don	800	308
30	Boggia	Bart	800	308

SHW = Super heavyweight

800-lb Deadlift Club

Rank	Last name	First Name	Lift (lbs)	Weight class
1	Harold	Tim	855	SHW
2	Smith	Matt	850	SHW
3	Anderson	Jake	845	308
4	Edwards	Luke	840	275
5	Vogelpohl	Chuck	835	275
6	Stafford	John	832	275
7	Hoff	Dave	825	275
8	Dimel	Matt	821	SHW
9	Ruggiera	Mike	821	SHW
10	Panora	Greg	815	242
11	Obradovic	Jerry	810	308
12	Alhazov	Vlad	805	SHW

Rank	Last name	First Name	Lift (lbs)	Weight class
13	Meyers	Jeremiah	805	275
14	Holdsworth	JL	804	275
15	Brown	Mike	804	308
16	Paulucci	Tom	800	275
17	Douglas	Rich	800	275

SHW = Super heavyweight

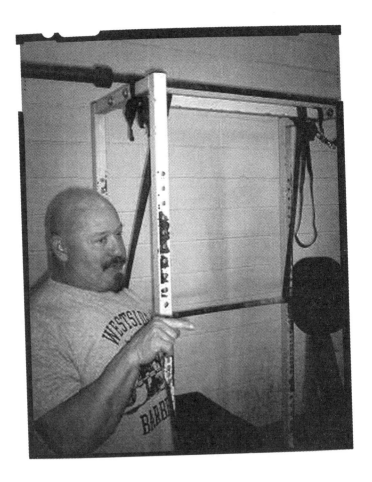

ABOUT THE AUTHOR

Louie Simmons is a strength coach, author, inventor, and lecturer. He has authored over 100 strength articles and three books and holds six U.S. patents. He has been the most innovative trainer in the last sixty years and is known throughout the world. Louie made a top ten lift in all three lifts and total from 1972–2002—a span of thirty years. His training methods have stood and will stand the test of time.

B esides Westside Barbell's 88 elite totals, Louie's expertise has produced bigger squats and deadlifts all over the world. His unique way of thinking and assistance has also helped MMA fighters, track and field athletes, and football players raise their performance to a whole new level.